ARE ALIENS MAKING
YOU FAT?

*The Surprising Truth about Your Weight Gain
from a Nutritional Expert and Amateur Alienologist.*

DR. SCOTT OLSON ND

What I love about the modern world (except for the aliens) is that a book is no longer just a book. I invite you to join the fun on my website www.thealiendiet.com where you can sign up for an online class that guides you through the diet section of this book. Each e-mail has a daily discussion, three recipes (for over 100 new recipes), a daily challenge and links for further reading and much more!

As with any diet, I strongly encourage you to work with your local medical professional before making any changes to your diet. If you follow the recommendations in this book, your blood sugar will change and this can be dangerous if you are already on medications.

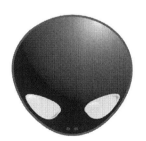

ISBN-10: 1452849366
EAN-13: 9781452849362

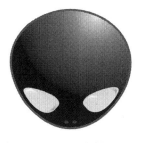

INTRODUCTION

You probably don't lie awake at night thinking about the state of human health and nutrition, but I do.

The word "geek" is usually reserved for people who love math, science, or other technical pursuits, but a geek is exactly what I am. My geekiness, though, is reserved for exploring what we as humans should be eating and uncovering the exact components of perfect human nutrition.

I've been studying health and nutrition my whole life (well… at least my whole *adult* life) and I have read more research papers on the subject of human health than is generally safe to admit to the boys while watching a Friday night basketball game. But while some people call my nutritional studies a bit overblown, my obsession with optimum human nutrition recently paid off; let me tell you about it.

One night, I was lying in my bed (geeking out) thinking about the Classic Puzzles of Human Nutrition, when a new thought came to me: Could all of the nutritional puzzles somehow be connected? While dietary conundrums are something I think about daily, I'm guessing that you have never heard of anything as strange as a "classic nutritional puzzle." While you may have never heard of them, they are probably something with which you are familiar; take a look:

- **Most people lose weight only to gain it back again** (this alone should make you think something otherworldly is going on around here). This yo-yo dieting is so common that almost everyone over the age of eighteen has experienced it some time in their lives.
- **Health fads change with every year.** Today it is a low-carb diet that will make you skinny; next year it is high-protein diet; and the year after that it is the banana, peppermint tea, and grapefruit diet. These fad diets maybe work for a little while, but then they stop and the pounds return to your hips and thighs.
- **Myths trump facts.** The facts about what you should be eating are lost in a sea of myths about nutrition. In fact, you are taught many health myths in school (such as milk is essential for your bones and you must eat a large amount of protein to be healthy). While you have outgrown the need for Santa Claus, leprechauns, and the Easter Bunny, you still cling to these misunderstandings about what your body truly needs to thrive.
- **People shun foods that are good for them.** How many people have you heard say that they don't like the taste of donuts? Now compare that number to the number of people who say that they don't like broccoli, or salad greens, or carrots, or even apples and pears. How is it that our taste buds are magnetized to foods that are no good for us?

And the most puzzling nutritional puzzle of them all: **Despite that fact that we are in a position to feed ourselves better than humans have ever been fed, we don't.** We can eat summer foods in winter; we have refrigeration and other means of preserving our food for which previous generations of humans would have killed. The varieties of foods that we can eat every day were simply not available to our ancestors. We should be the skinniest and healthiest creatures on the planet, but somehow we are not.

What makes these puzzles even more puzzling is that human scientists who do research are *not* confused about what we should be eating. Our scientists know exactly what we should be putting in our mouths if we want to lose weight and be healthy. And it is not just our scientists who all agree on what we should be eating. The World Health Organization, The American Heart Association, The American Diabetes Association, and countless other groups now say that somewhere between 70 and 90 percent of all illnesses can be avoided through proper nutrition. Yes, you read that correctly: 70 to 90 percent of all the illnesses we encounter (including being overweight) are the direct results of the food and lifestyle choices we make every day.

Are you starting to see what keeps me up at night wondering what in the world is going on? On one hand, most of us believe that we can eat whatever we want and still be healthy, but on the other hand nutritional scientists understand that we need to focus on certain foods if we want to stay slim and healthy. Which is right?

Recently I was standing in line at the supermarket reading magazine covers and noticed that one article claimed that I could lose up to two pounds of fat a day while not changing what I eat at all; another article suggested that I could lose weight while I sleep. And yet, there are large scientific population studies, including *The China Study* and the *Framingham Heart Study*, that suggest what you eat matters not only to your waistline, but also to your health and longevity.

Why is there such a gap between what we know and what our scientists know? That is the exact question I was asking myself that night when I was lying in bed puzzling over my favorite nutritional quandaries. It was then that I began to become suspicious that there was something strange going on, something that was so powerful that it invaded every aspect of our lives and yet no one knew about it. It was in that half-awake, half-asleep time that I had a dream. In the dream I was a rat living in a scientist's lab. The other rats and I were being fed foods that were making us sick, but we behaved as if everything was normal. We had no idea that we were being used as an experiment for someone else's needs.

The dream was so startling that I sat up when I realized what it meant. The nutritional puzzles that had mystified me for years all suddenly made complete sense. I used to think that the nutritional puzzles were separate, but what if they were all connected? What if someone (or something) was performing experiments on us? What if we were rats in some scientist's lab? That was silly, I thought; no one could pull off such a colossal nutritional hoax on the whole of humanity. But the thought wouldn't leave me and the questions continued: If someone was manipulating us, what would be the point of that kind of experiment?

Then it hit me: There was only one answer to all those questions and that was that alien scientists were experimenting on the whole human race. It must be aliens who were pulling our nutritional strings. It had to be aliens because they would be the only ones who could mastermind and coordinate such a huge effort. Okay, I admit it sounds a bit crazy that aliens are using us as lab rats (as it did to me when I first thought of it), but wait until you read more.

The first stop is a visit to a rat's cage.

THE RAT'S PERSPECTIVE

Take a moment to imagine what it might be like if you were a rat living in some scientist's lab (like in my dream).

Every morning you wake up, stretch, and scratch behind your ears. You then start your morning ritual: You say good morning to the other rats in your neighborhood and then head over to your bowl to get a drink. After hydrating yourself, you hop on your exercise wheel for a bit of exercise. You might eat a bit, explore your cage, and then you lie down for a nap.

The rest of your day is pretty much the same: eat, exercise, rest, and repeat. Now that you are comfy with your rat lifestyle, let me ask you a question: What do you think is normal for a rat? You were born in a cage and you have lived every day of your life in that cage; as you look around, all the rats you know are living in cages that look exactly like yours. Every one of your rat friends has the same setup: a nice little home with a soft bed, all the food they could want, and a wheel for exercising. From time to time a human pulls you out your cage and weighs you, or takes your blood, or has you run a maze, but this is happening to everyone around you so you think it must be normal. Again, let me ask you a question: Do you know you are part of some experiment?

No, you think that *this must be how all rats live.* After all, this life is all you have ever known. A rat in a scientist's cage knows nothing about how rats are really supposed to live. Even though everyone in the rat neighborhood is getting fat, or has cancer, diabetes, or is having little rat heart attacks, they are mostly content with their lives. They get enough food, have a good place to sleep, and someone else cleans up their cages.

This little thought experiment points out the difficulty we have with looking around us to decide what is normal; your eyes lie to you. If you were to ask a rat what she thinks is normal, she would glance around and conclude that every rat in the world must live in plastic cages; she knows nothing of natural rat habitats (and everyone knows rats live in sewers and aboard pirate ships). The question you have to ask yourself is this: Are you a rat? If a rat in scientist's lab doesn't know what is normal and cannot trust her eyes to tell her the truth, maybe we can't either.

Think about it. Most humans you encounter are eating exactly what you are eating and they are living a life very similar to yours. But no animal alive today or at any time in the history of this planet has eaten the way that you do, or lived the way that you do. Everywhere you look, people are eating highly processed foods full of sugar, salt, and fat, but is that really normal for humans? People are living lives of high stress and not taking time to exercise, relax, or to connect with people they love; is that that the way we should be living?

Your diet may seem normal to you; your neighbors go to the same stores and eat at the same restaurants that you do. But if you want to discover just how abnormal your diet is, all you have to do is hop in a plane (or a time machine) to discover that the fast-food-prepackaged-artificially-injected-instant-pretend foods that make it to your plate every day are a modern-day monstrosity only available to those lucky enough to afford this lifetime of obesity and illness.

This is the thought that jolted me out of bed: Could we all be just like a rat in some crazy experiment? But as soon as I thought it, I quickly put it out of my mind because no one on earth could pull off such a crazy experiment. I also couldn't figure out what would be the point of such an experiment (until later). The foods that people are eating are making them fat and unhealthy; what group on earth would want such a thing?

There are plenty of villains at whom you could point your finger who might benefit from steering us down the nutritional road to our doom. Maybe doctors and the medical establishment want to have a steady stream of patients so they give you bad advice about your diet (or give you no advice at all). Or maybe food manufacturers only want to make foods that are tasty and addictive to increase their income and boost their stock prices. Maybe governments don't want to pay our Social Security, so they benefit from giving people bad advice that will shorten their lives.

None of that made any sense. After all, it is your teachers telling you that milk is good for you; it is your mother baking those cookies; it is your friends handing you the soda and that bag of potato chips; it is your government suggesting that sugar is not harmful.[1] Your teachers, your mother, and your friends are all humans and they wouldn't knowingly cause you harm. It was then that the realization came to me: If no one on earth could pull off such a dietary hoax, then the answer had to be otherworldly.

The evidence is simple: If I were to design a diet and a lifestyle that could cause the most harm to human beings, I would develop a diet that is exactly what you are eating right now: a diet high in fat, protein, sugar, salt, and preservatives and low in fresh fruits and vegetables. The diet that most people eat is designed to cater to their taste buds (and to alien agendas), but not what their bodies need to thrive.

We have all been tricked, but you can fight back against this nutritional onslaught.

YOU THE ALIEN

Let's stop pretending that we are rats in a cage and switch our imagination game to the other side of the galaxy to take a look inside the brains of the aliens who are experimenting with your life.

---

1   The Dietary Reference Intake Reports of the National Academy of Sciences Food and Nutrition boards currently suggests that not more than 25 percent of your total calories should come from added sugars. That means that one-quarter of everything you eat can be white sugar.

Imagine that you are now an alien and that you have far superior technology than we do. You have lots of advanced technology, but your people are still not healthy and you want to find out why. Since you are an alien scientist, you know that you should do experiments to understand how different diets might affect health, but experimenting on your own people is just too hard and not ethical. So you look around the universe and discover a race of beings called "humans" on a planet called "earth." These humans are just close enough to your own physiology to be great test subjects for your health experiments (this similar to the way we use rats, even though they are different species).

These humans are perfect test subjects, you think and you then hatch a plan to have humans eat a diet you suspect would cause disease in any animal you could trick into eating it. The funny thing is that you don't really have to work that hard because humans will eat anything that is salty, fatty, and sweet. To make your plan really work, why don't you make sure that humans think they even *need* some of the very foods that harm them by having so-called nutritional experts, government agencies, and even schools support your evil plans? If you don't think this type of manipulation of our society is possible, then try this quick mini-quiz:

- What food should you eat to build strong bones?
- What food is high in potassium?
- If you want strong muscles, what do you eat?

If you answered milk, bananas, and protein to the above questions then you are already under the influence of the evil alien's spell and are simply repeating the messages that they put into your head. All of those messages, by the way, are wrong (but we can talk about that later).

Okay, back to your alien homeland: Your superior alien intelligence also helps you to realize another key to your plan is to make the foods you want humans to eat cheap, fast, and easy to get a hold of and make the foods they should be eating expensive and harder to acquire.

Humans also tend to stay away from most foods that are good for them because they say they don't like the taste of them. You can laugh your evil alien laugh at this point because (as you know) if humans feast on super-sweet, super-fat, and super-salty foods, then their taste buds lie to them and tell them that naturally good foods such as broccoli, cabbage, and kale don't taste good and even naturally sweet foods such as carrots, apples, and pears taste odd. It only takes a little while for your test subjects who are eating alien inspired foods to begin to shun real foods and only trust prepackaged nutritionally nonsensical foods you know will make them ill.

It also doesn't hurt your alien experimental plans that many of the foods you want humans to eat are also addicting. You may know that foods that contain caffeine are addictive, but other foods humans eat are also addictive, including chocolate, dairy, and (the especially powerful) sugary foods. These addictions, our human scientists are learning, are just as strong as addictions to alcohol and cigarettes and have health consequences just as severe.

The alien plan to experiment on humans by having them eat foods that make their taste buds happy, but destroy their bodies is all too easy. Soon the humans think that these laboratory-inspired foods are what they are supposed to eat (after all everyone is doing it).

WHAT'S FOR BREAKFAST?

Let's take a minute to talk about the human animal: We certainly are funny and interesting creatures. What seems to set humans apart from many creatures is our big brain, but that brain can get us into all sorts of trouble – especially at the breakfast table.

You don't see a cow wondering what it should eat; his breakfast is right under his feet. Likewise, a lion doesn't worry too much about its choice of a meal; it is that animal running right in front of her. Think about the effort it takes to determine what foods we should be eating. We scrutinize labels on the back of packaged foods, trying to determine whether they are all right to give to our families; our scientists spend countless hours and billions of dollars trying to uncover the secrets to long life; and we try fad diets hoping to unlock the key to weight loss. The absurdity of picking up a book to tell you what you should be eating is an experience unique to humans and humans alone (but something that may be necessary because aliens are influencing what is going in our mouths).

Humans have wandered far from our own pastures. Imagine a cow that finds herself surrounded by nothing but streets. Looking around, she sees other cows eating and licking the ground; thinking that is normal, she too starts eating the black asphalt. That is the exact place we find ourselves today: eating poison and thinking it is normal.

Eating the way that we eat is not without its repercussions. There are consequences to eating alien foods that are far more insidious than just that extra weight you may be carrying around. Our diets lead us down a path towards an unhappy destination: poor health, dependence on medications, obesity, and shortened lives. The way you are eating is not only increasing your weight, it is also depriving you of a long life and increasing the number of visits you will make to your medical doctor's office.

Whether nutritional puzzles puzzle you like they do me or not, you have to admit that something strange is going on around here. You and I have the opportunity to feed ourselves better than any humans have ever been fed, and yet we shovel non-foods into our mouths every day that only make us sicker and fatter.

You might be thinking I'm a bit crazy for suggesting that aliens are controlling our diets (and you might be right), but what is even more crazy is thinking that it is humans who are responsible for this nutritional titanic we are all sailing on. Why would a race of beings develop a diet that is only going to shorten their time on this earth? It seems crazy that human corporations would produce foods that lead to disease, or that governments, teachers, and medical professionals would support this nutritional nonsense. The only thing that makes sense (because surely human companies and human institutions are looking out for our best interests) is that aliens are somehow manipulating our diets.

I blame aliens. I blame aliens for getting us into this mess. I blame aliens for the fact that we are getting fatter, getting sicker, and living half-lives because we are sicker and fatter. I blame aliens for making us think that we need to count calories, or assign points to every food that we eat, or that we need to spend large sums of money to lose weight. We don't.

Who knows what the aliens are really up to: Maybe they are experimenting on humans by manipulating our diet; or maybe they are just planning to take over the world and their invasion plans would go much easier if we are all too fat or too sick to fight them; or maybe the aliens have discovered the easiest way to destroy humans is simply let them do it to themselves. All I know is that when I look around at the foods we are eating, they are not the foods that we should be eating.

These aliens have to be stopped and they have to be stopped right now, but to fight aliens you are going to need a plan. As luck would have it, I've uncovered what makes the aliens plan work so fiendishly well and what you can do about it.

YOUR BATTLE PLAN

You are going to need an action plan if you are going to fight aliens (and I'll provide you with a specific one later in the book), but let me run some ideas by you right now so you understand what is required of you if you are going to get out from under the influence of aliens and their alien food.

Most of what you have read up to this point has been about your health (well, that and evil aliens); I have yet to mention much about weight loss. There are good reasons for this and it ends up being the most important thing you can learn from this book, so pay attention.

In these times of danger (for not only you but the whole human race) you have to stop thinking that health and weight loss are separate things.

Your health and good weight management are the same thing. In fact, drop the notion of losing weight right now and turn your focus on your health because (as you shall see) when you become healthier, you will lose all the weight you want.

Here is the big secret that the aliens don't want you to know: Your body *wants* to be at a healthy weight, but it is not going to give you what you want until you give your body what it needs. What does your body need? That is the million-dollar question and the subject of the rest of this book. While you might think that there is a lot of debate about what constitutes a healthy diet for humans, there actually is no debate at all (or at least much less than you would think). The reason you might be confused about what you should be eating is simple: Aliens are keeping you from the truth.

Over one half off our population is now considered overweight or obese. Do you think this might have something to do with what we are putting in our mouths? Our human scientists estimate that changing the way you eat can lead to a much longer and healthier life. What our scientists are collectively saying is that the hundreds of small choices that you make every day about what you eat are not trivial; they all have an impact on your life and well-being.

Eating better can improve not only your weight and your health, but also your longevity. Longevity is nice, but who wants to live longer if they can't enjoy their lives? That is what being healthier offers you: not only more days on the earth, but much *better* days on the earth.

When people take care of themselves and eat better they are less likely to have crippling diseases such as diabetes, heart disease, arthritis, osteoporosis, Alzheimer's, and even cancer. That means that they are less likely to have to walk around needing things like oxygen tanks, wheelchairs, heart monitors, or having to wear diapers when they get old. Changing the way you eat today means that you won't be following all your neighbors down the pathway to ill health and an ever-growing list of medications and medical procedures you need just to stay alive. No, changing your lifestyle means that you are putting yourself down a different path than the rest of your neighbors, one full of energy, health, vibrancy, and the weight you want.

This is no small matter. Atkins, South Beach, Weight Watchers, Mediterranean, Grapefruit, and so many other diets fail you because they are not giving your body what it needs. Yes, you will lose weight on these diets. But are you healthier after you have followed one of these diets? The answer is no.

Humans are meant to eat a large amount of the very foods that the aliens don't want them to eat: vegetables and fruits. Aliens think that you are not smart enough to realize their evil plan; even if you do, they think that you will never make the transition from fake foods to real foods because you are weak and pathetic creatures. I think differently.

You don't have to go out and buy a space-ray gun to do battle with aliens; you simply have to change what you are doing every day and the aliens will lose interest in you as a test subject. Yes, you can do battle with aliens without leaving your home. While this might sound crazy right now, fighting aliens can be as simple as eating more broccoli.

Let's take a look.

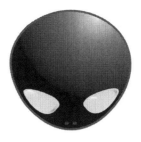

ALIEN RECIPES

Before we look at how you can do battle with aliens and how you can turn the tide on this nutritional nightmare that we all find ourselves in, let's take a look to see how we got here. When we understand what the aliens are doing to make us fat means, then we also understand what we need to do to change it.

Like anybody who cooks, aliens have recipes that have been perfected over time. These recipes are not for dinner, though; they are for making humans fat and sick. The aliens have five different components to their *Make Humans Fat* recipe. Here they are:

1. Eat sugars and foods that act like sugars.
2. Eat a large amount of the wrong kinds of fats.
3. Become addicted to food that is unhealthy.
4. Shun vegetables and fruits.
5. Refuse to move their bodies around.

Let's take a look at each of these and see how they are contributing to our weight gain and general well-being.

SUGARS

The first ingredient for making humans fat and sick is sugar.

We have all sorts of ways to describe the joy that sugar brings us. The word "sweet" is used in our language for foods that taste sweet, but it is also used when we describe people we like and loved ones. Think about these words: sweetie, sugar, and honey. They are all used to tell someone we love them (see how tricky the aliens are?). But while sugar sounds and tastes enjoyable, it also has a dark side. Sugar destroys our bodies. There is a part of you that knows how bad sugar can be for your health, so while you might crave it you have a gut feeling that you shouldn't be eating as much of the white stuff as you do.

Most people know that cutting sugars out of their diet can have a dramatic effect on their weight. If you have ever tried a low-carb diet, you know that they work. The creators of the South Beach, Atkins, and other low-carb diets got part of the weight-loss equation correct: Sugars do pile on the fat and removing them from your diet leads to weight loss. The problem with low-carb diets is that they forgot one little thing: Fat also adds weight and, more importantly, eating a high-fat diet has the potential to dramatically shorten your life. More on that subject later; let's keep talking about sugars.

A TON OF SUGAR

People generally have no idea how much sugar goes into their mouths every day. I've written a book on sugar, called *Sugarettes*, which goes into detail about how sugars are addictive and harmful so I won't talk too much about it here, but let's go over the main points.

Current estimates are that each person in the United States (and other Western countries) consumes somewhere around 150 to 170 pounds of sugar every year. If you pull out your handy calculator and hit the divide button you realize that you are eating around half a pound of sugar every day of your life.

If you are shaking your head right now, wondering how you can eat that much sugar in a day, let's take a look from where that sugar is coming. The first thing you need to know is that a pound of sugar is equal to 120 teaspoons. Now let's look at how much sugar can be found in common foods:

- One twelve-ounce soda contains 8 teaspoons of sugar.
- Donuts contain 8-10 teaspoons of sugar.
- Jams contain 3 teaspoons per tablespoon.
- Cookies have 2-4 teaspoons per cookie.

Soda is, by far, the biggest source of added sugars in our lives; after all, who drinks only twelve ounces at a time? Most restaurants serve at least a sixteen-ounce drink (with free refills) and if you decide to drop by the Quickie Mart and pick up one of those Super 42-ounce sodas, that soda alone contains one-quarter pound of sugar.

But our sugar gorging doesn't stop there: your morning cereal, your Starbucks coffee drink, your chips, your afternoon snack; they all have sugar in them. Add to that the so-called "hidden sugars" found in salad dressings, sauces, breads, peanut butter, ketchup, and in almost every other food we eat. But it is not just the white sugar or added sugar for which you have to look out; it is also the foods that act like sugars in your body (more on that later). Most people don't believe that they are eating a half-pound of sugar every day. It is actually very easy to eat your daily ration of sugar (what is hard is the opposite: not eating that much sugar).

What the modern alien-inspired sugar-world is doing, in a sense, is creating a grand scientific experiment with your body. Take your body (that thrives on basic foods such as fruits and vegetables) and feed it highly refined sugars and carbohydrates and see what happens. The result of this experiment is that we have more heart disease, more diabetes, more cancer, and more people with excessive weight walking around.

The problem with too much sugar in our bodies is twofold. The first is that sugar makes the cells in our bodies less sensitive to insulin (the hormone that controls blood sugar). Less sensitive cells are a condition called "insulin insensitivity," which is a step towards diabetes. The second problem our sweet friend creates is that sugar is easily converted into fat inside our bodies.

Let's take a look at both of these problems.

INSULIN INSENSITIVITY

One of the major problems with having a large amount of sugar running around in your blood all the time is that the cells in your body change from being responsive to insulin to being not responsive to insulin. The reason your cells stop responding to insulin is that when there is a large amount of sugar in your bloodstream there is also a large amount of insulin (the hormone your body uses to control your blood sugar). Insulin works like a key to a door, which opens up the cell and allows sugar inside. It works like this: When there is sugar in your bloodstream, insulin "knocks" on the cell's door; the cell opens the door and sugar goes into the cell. The problem is that cells only need so much sugar and get tired of the constant knocking on their door, so if there is a lot of insulin in the blood, they start ignoring insulin's knock. This so-called "insulin insensitivity" is a pre-diabetic state. In fact, diabetes is an extreme form of insulin insensitivity, in which the cells almost ignore insulin knocking completely.

Why is it bad that cells are ignoring insulin's knock? Remember that it is insulin's job to move sugar from the bloodstream into the cells; when the cells of the body become insensitive to insulin that means the sugar that would normally go into your cells is now just floating around in your bloodstream. A bloodstream full of sugar is a problem for your body because it now has to do something with all that extra sugar. The solution is to store that sugar as fat (see the next section).

And here is the really crazy thing about all of this: The more body fat you have, the more insulin insensitivity you have. You can probably already tell that this whole cycle is a terrible endless loop: insulin insensitivity creates more weight gain, which creates more insulin insensitivity, which creates more weight gain, which... you get the idea.

SUGAR INTO FAT

Sugar's second evil quality is that it is easily converted into fat. We have talked a little bit about this above, but let's take a closer look at how this happens. Watch what happens when you eat something that contains a carbohydrate and follow a molecule of sugar (called glucose) from the time you eat it all the way to your hips. It doesn't matter if this sugar molecule comes from table sugar, grains, pasta, syrup, or any other carbohydrate, to your body it is all the same. Remember this: Sugars come in many forms, but to your body they are all the same.

Our story starts when you take a bite of that birthday cake, drink a soda, or eat potato chips. That carbohydrate enters your stomach for digestion. Your digestive system will break down all the complex sugars in that cake, soda, or chips into simple sugars (like glucose) and soon those molecules of glucose find their way from your stomach into your bloodstream.

Having sugar in your bloodstream is no problem; in fact, your body needs glucose to run all its bodily functions. If you ate whole, plant-based foods, your blood sugar would rise slowly and never get too high. The problem arises if you eat a large amount of simple sugars or foods that act like sugars in your body (which most people do). When you eat like a typical American, you dump a large amount of sugar into your bloodstream all day long.

Your body, like your tongue, really likes sugar (this is one of the reasons why we crave it so much). Glucose, one of the basic units of energy, can be used as fuel in your body for many things. The problem is that your body can only use so much sugar before it has enough fuel to meet all its needs. Once the body has those needs met, the problems start. The body now has a bunch of extra energy (in the form of glucose) floating around and it needs to find something to do with that extra fuel.

Your body is not stupid; it doesn't want to waste that cake-energy you have just eaten because it knows that wasting is not a good idea. Your body is going to want to keep that energy around, so it stores that extra sugar as—yes, you guessed it—fat.

Remember, that for most of human history, there would be times when food was easy to acquire and other times when it was hard. Your body wants to store that energy in case there is a time when there is not enough food around. When you eat a bunch of sugar your body is smart to store that energy in your tummy, or waist, or hips, waiting for the day (that never comes to our modern world) when there is not enough food around.

Now also remember that for the bulk of human history the foods we ate never caused such a large spike in our blood sugar. The foods that you eat today are not the foods your ancestors ate. The high sugar meal is a modern invention (one might even suspect that it was devised by aliens).

This is the story of how a sugary meal gets turned into fat in your body. Glucose makes its way from your mouth to your stomach and then it takes a trip to your thighs, waiting for the day you need it (that often never comes). The first key to battling aliens, then, is to keep blood sugar under more control. But how do you keep your blood sugar low? That is simple: stay away from all sugars and foods that act like sugars.

What are the foods that act like sugars? I'm glad you asked.

FOODS THAT ACT LIKE SUGARS

While you might think that eating a half-pound of sugar is a lot every day (and it is), but the story gets even worse because most people don't realize that many foods that they eat every day act just like sugar in their bodies.

If you had a magic blood sugar monitor you could strap to your wrist that would instantly tell you what your blood sugar was throughout the day, you would notice that it makes very little difference to your body when you drink a soda or eat some French bread. To your body, French bread and soda are the same: They both cause your blood sugar to increase dramatically.

The reason we know that French bread (and other foods) cause your blood sugar to rise just like sugar is because of the work of David Jenkins, MD, PhD, a professor of nutrition at the University of Toronto. For years we thought certain foods kept blood sugar low and others raised blood sugar, but we never tested our theory. Dr. Jenkins had the novel idea of feeding people individual foods and then seeing what those foods did to blood sugar. The result of his (and other scientist's) research is what we now call the glycemic index. The glycemic index is a measurement of how individual foods are expected to change our blood sugar when we eat them. What we have discovered is that there are many foods that act more like sugar in our bodies than white sugar does. Yes, some foods increase our blood sugar more than eating white sugar does.

What these studies have found is that there are high glycemic index foods (foods that really increase blood sugar) and low glycemic index foods (those that change our blood sugar only a little) and everything in between.

Take a look at the glycemic index values for these common foods:

White Rice	111
Pancakes	104
Glucose	100
Rice Cakes	91
Corn Flakes	92
Wonder Bread	71
Sucrose (table sugar)	64

The numbers in the glycemic index are not important; you just need to know that the higher the number the higher your blood sugar goes. As you can see, to your body, it makes no difference if you have eaten straight glucose (sugar) or pancakes, the results are the same: high blood sugar. The glycemic index can be complex and depends a lot on the character of the individual food. You can find web-based glycemic index charts if you want to explore the concept a little bit more.

The glycemic index can be summed up with this chart:

High Glycemic Foods	Sugar (of course), any refined grain-based food (think: breads, chips, donuts, cereals...) cooked potatoes (French fries...) and a few fruits (bananas, watermelon...).
Medium Glycemic Foods	Whole grains eaten as whole grains (like rice, barley, but not whole grain breads), some beans, pasta.
Low Glycemic Foods	Most fruits and vegetables (but not potato), proteins (like fish, chicken, beef), nuts

The reason it is important to know about the foods that act like sugars is so you can understand that it does no good to stay away from sugars if you don't take into account that there are many foods that act exactly like white sugar in your body. If your goal is weight loss, one of the keys to that weight loss has to be to keep your blood sugar low—and that means staying away from both sugars and foods that act like sugars. But don't cause yourself too much trouble by trying to determine the glycemic index of everything you eat; there is an easier way.

The best way to eat low-glycemic foods is to make sure your plate is full of whole, unprocessed foods. Don't worry that potatoes, bananas, or watermelons are high on the glycemic index, as long as they are surrounded by a large amount of other vegetables in your diet. I'll have more to say about just what you should be eating later in the book. For now, just remember: Whole, unprocessed foods are generally low on the glycemic index.

NATURAL SUGARS ARE NO DIFFERENT

At this point you may be thinking that it is time to ditch the sugars and the foods that act like sugars, but you still would like to have something sweet. The next question that usually pops into people's heads is, "Can I have honey, maple syrup, agave, or other natural sugar?" I hate to disappoint you, but the answer is no.

While honey, agave, and some other so-called "natural" sugars are lower on the glycemic index, they still are 100-percent sugars. Most of these natural sugars contain a high amount of fructose (which may be much worse than glucose). Fructose in your blood is much more likely to lead to insulin insensitivity than glucose and it is also more likely to be stored as fat (remember, more fat is what you *don't* want).

It is true that honey and real maple syrup do contain some small amount of minerals and other nutrients, but the amounts of these minerals are so small and not worth the burden that eating these sugars places on your body.

ARTIFICIAL SWEETENERS

If you are still looking for something sweet, artificial sweeteners are no place to turn either. These man-made chemicals don't belong in your body and have been associated with numerous health issues. We normally talk about the side effects of drugs, but artificial sweeteners also have side effects that range from headaches, to diarrhea, to neurological (nerve) problems, and to a host of other symptoms. [1] Aspartame alone was once the most complained about food additives on the planet.[2]

Many of these artificial sweeteners have been linked to diseases. Saccharine may cause bladder cancer and aspartame is broken down in the body to methanol (a known toxin), which has been linked to many diseases.

Artificial sweeteners not only destroy your health, but they also don't help you to lose weight. Yes, you read that right. You turn to the artificial sweeteners to avoid weight gain and guess what happens? You don't lose weight. I have yet to read one study that suggests that consuming artificial sweeteners helps you lose weight. This is a bit strange considering that the reason people consume this junk is to help them lose weight. There are, however, studies that show the opposite. You eat these fake sugars and you can actually gain weight. It has been shown that the use of artificial sweeteners can actually cause you to consume *more* calories than if you weren't eating them in the first place.[3] The reason artificial sweeteners may cause you to overeat is not clear, but it may be enough to understand that your body does not like to be tricked. Artificial sweeteners fool your body into believing that you are going to be eating something sweet, but you are not.

The worst part of using artificial sweeteners is that they continue your addiction to unnaturally sweet tastes. If you go on a diet that removes all super-sweet foods from your life, you will find that your taste buds adapt and you enjoy a more subtle sweetness found in all sorts of healthy foods.

WHAT ABOUT STEVIA?

Okay, I can't find much bad to say about Stevia, but it still sits on my caution list. Stevia is a plant that is super sweet and Stevia extracts can be found in health food stores. Stevia actually helps to balance blood sugar and contains no calories. The only thing I would caution you with about eating Stevia is that using it will continue your addiction to sweet-tasting foods.

Consider using Stevia as a transition sweetener or for occasional use.

Summing it all up

Here is what you want to remember about sugar:

- You are eating a ton of sugar (whether you know it or not).

- Eating a large amount of sugar is a steps towards diabetes (whether doctors know it or not).

- Sugar turns into fat (whether you like it or not).

- But it is not just white sugar you have to look out for, remember that there are foods that act like sugars (these are the high glycemic foods) and honey, agave, maple syrup and other so-called natural syrups act just like white sugar in your body.

- If you are looking for a sweetener, stay away from artificial sweeteners but if you absolutely need a sweetener, give Stevia a try.

THE FAT PROBLEM

The second ingredient in the alien's "Make the Humans Fat" stew is, well, fat. Seems to make sense, doesn't it? Eating too much fat makes you fat. The problem is that when most people think about fat, they think about foods like butter and oils, but there is a huge source of fat that you might be overlooking (I told you those aliens are tricky).

Fats pose three problems to your continued good health. The first is that fats contain more calories per gram than any other foods and that means that they can easily add to your waistline. The second is that eating certain types of fats is associated with an increase in blood cholesterol (and all the problems that come with that). The third problem is that a high-fat diet is directly associated with many diseases that we see every day attacking our loved ones, including heart disease, diabetes, Alzheimer's, and cancer.

We'll take a closer look at the sources of fat in your diet and what you can do about it, but let's first take a closer look at why fats are so harmful to human beings.

FAT MATH

Remember what you read in the previous pages about sugar and how sugars get turned into fat in our bodies? Too much sugar in your bloodstream leads the liver to process those extra sugar energy molecules into fat. What I didn't tell you was that the conversion of sugars into fat takes energy. Typically, you burn about 23 percent of the energy in sugar to convert glucose (sugar) into fat. This means that if you ate a one hundred-calorie meal of just sugar, you would burn twenty-three of those calories in order to store that energy as fat. So, you one-hundred-calorie meal becomes only seventy-seven calories worth of fat on your body (still not great, but it is good to know that you are burning something in order to make that conversion).

Now, imagine a food from which you don't have to spend any energy to convert it into fat. Imagine a meal where you ate one hundred calories and it ended up as one hundred calories of fat on your body. This magic food—you guessed it—is our old friend the fat molecule. If you consume one hundred calories of fat, your body needs only three calories to move the fat from your meal to fat on your belly, butt, chin, and thighs. That means that with every one hundred calories of fat that you consume, there is the potential to add ninety-seven calories of fat to your bottom and your bottom line.

But the story of fat gets even worse. Let's take a look.

FAT CALORIES

Now, while you are contemplating how easy it is for your body to convert fat in food to fat on your body, think about this: Fat contains more calories than any other food. Take a look:

- Protein contains four calories per gram
- Carbohydrates contain four calories per gram
- Fat contains nine calories per gram

That means that for every gram of fat you eat, you are consuming the energy equivalent of more than twice that of proteins or carbohydrates. But I don't want you to get fat phobic; the news about fat isn't all bad. Fat serves many essential purposes in our bodies:

- Many of our hormones are built upon cholesterol molecule.
- Fat is also our insulation system, helping us to keep warm.
- Fat forms part of our brains and nervous systems.
- Fats help carry vitamins throughout our bodies.
- Fat is also our backup energy system. Should our bodies ever run out of fuel, this stored energy is then released into our bloodstream and converted back into glucose (sugar).

The problem with this last point is that most people never get to the fat-burning stage. If you were a free human living in the wild, far away from alien influences, you would put fat on your body when food was abundant, but then burn it off when it was not. In your current rat-in-the-cage lifestyle, you never get to the "burning the fat off" stage. The big question for the seeker of a trimmer waistline is: How do you get to the fat-burning stage? The simple and short answer is that you need to turn your body into a fat-burning machine (but we will talk more about that later).

What is the take-home message here? Fats are extremely energy-dense foods and should only be used in small amounts. Now we should talk about which types of fats we are eating.

KNOW YOUR FATS

Not all fats are created equal, and if you are going to do battle with aliens, you need to know how they are different.

- **Cholesterol**: We hear a lot about cholesterol. It isn't technically a fat but a fat-like or waxy substance that can be found in animal products; your liver can also make it. Cholesterol is important for our bodies to make vitamin D and hormones. It can be found in large amounts in eggs, fish, meat, and dairy products (including butter).

After cholesterol, we divide fats up into four categories:

- **Monounsaturated fats** are fats found in plant sources such as avocados, olive oil, and nut and seed oils (peanut, sunflower, safflower, olive, and grapeseed oils).
- **Polyunsaturated fats** are fats in seed and nut oils, but also include fish oils and flax. Polyunsaturated fats can also be found in leafy green veggies and beans.
- **Saturated fats** are fats found almost exclusively in animal products, such as dairy (butter, cheese, cream, ice cream, yogurt), eggs, and meats (fish, chicken, red meats). There are saturated fats found in coconut and palm oils, but

these medium-chain saturated fats act differently in your body that the ones found in animal products.

- **Trans fats and Hydrogenated oils** are fats that are not found in any large amounts in nature and are totally alien to our bodies. Hydrogenated fats are created when liquid fats are made into solid fats (like margarine) by adding more hydrogen to the plant fat molecules. Trans fats are formed when fats are heated and when they are hydrogenated. These fats, we are learning, are harmful to our health, especially our hearts[4] and can be found in all manner of processed foods, including cookies, donuts, fast foods, crackers, margarine, and shortening.

If you want to spoil the alien's plan to make you a laboratory experiment, you need to stay away from the last two types of fats (saturated fats and the trans fats) and use the mono- and polyun-saturated fats sparingly.

FATTY DISEASES

Fat in our diet causes many problems. The most visible sign of consuming too much fat is that you gain weight, but the problems with a fatty diet go far beyond just how you look. Let's take a look at the common diseases associated with a high-fat diet:

- Prostate disease[5]
- Heart disease, including hypertension[6]
- Poor sugar control (metabolic syndrome)[7,8]
- Brain problems, including memory and cognitive performance[9]
- A high fat diet increases the risk of breast cancer. This is probably due to higher circulating hormone levels that come with a high fat diet.[10] It also may be a long-term effect; the sooner a girl switches to a low fat/high plant based diet, the better[11]
- Trans fats also raise the risk of breast cancer,[12] and increase inflammation in the body[13]

In a strange twist that makes alien scientists giggle, eating a high-fat meal also increases the consumption of other food.[14] While you might think that fat helps you to feel full (and it can), eating a fatty meal also seems to increase the number of calories you eat in a day.

LET'S TALK CHOLESTEROL

We cannot finish talking about fat and our health without talking about cholesterol. People are often confused about their own cholesterol level and how it relates to the foods that they eat. You may know your own cholesterol level and have heard that you should keep it below 200 mg/dL, but that is not the whole story.

Yes, eating fatty foods and foods that have cholesterol in them can affect your own cholesterol levels,[15] but your liver also makes its own cholesterol. Before we get to how you can lower your cholesterol, let's take a look at what having a high blood cholesterol level means for your health:

- Cholesterol is bad for the heart (this you probably already know). You have a higher risk of heart disease when your cholesterol is over 200, but cholesterol's effects are not limited to clogging of our arteries; high cholesterol is also associated with stroke, peripheral vascular disease, and even high blood pressure.
- High cholesterol levels have also been linked to diabetes.[16]
- According to T. Colin Campbell, the author of the book *The China Study*, reducing blood cholesterol levels would reduce the number of cancers we have, including cancers of the rectum, colon, lung, breast brain, stomach, and esophagus, as well as adult and childhood leukemia.[17]

Perhaps the most astonishing information about cholesterol is a suggestion from Dr. William Castelli. While you probably have never heard his name, Dr. Castelli was the director of the world famous Framingham Heart Study (which you also probably have never heard of). The Framingham Study, which started in the 1940s, was initially started to investigate heart disease but has branched out and now includes other diseases.

What comes from studying people's heart health for over sixty years? Dr. Castelli suggests that not one person in the sixty years of study who had a cholesterol level below 150 mg/dL ever had a heart attack.[18] Think about that! You have the potential to reduce or eliminate the possibility of having a heart attack by simply changing the way that you eat. Another study, called The China Study, also showed that people with a cholesterol level below 150 were much healthier than people who had higher cholesterol levels.

Keeping your cholesterol below 150 may be your ticket, not only to weight loss, but also to a long and healthy life.

THE SOURCES OF FAT YOU MAY BE

OVERLOOKING

After reading everything above, you may be thinking that you should stay away from all fats and cholesterol, but that is not totally true. You should, though, make an effort to stay away most of the fats that find their way into your diet. While you should watch the obvious fats (such as butter and oils), you also have to look out for the sneaky fats in your diet that you may be overlooking. Where are those fats in your diet? Take a look:

- Dairy products, including milk and milk products, such as butter, yogurt, cheese
- Fake and Trans fats: Margarine, shortenings, cooking oils
- Animal products, including red meats, poultry, seafood, eggs, lard, and butter
- Fried food, including donuts, French fries, fried chicken...
- Eggs
- Nuts
- Salad dressing
- Mayonnaise

- Gravies
- Cooking oils
- Sauces

The largest sources of hidden fats are found in the animal proteins that we eat every day.

PROTEINS

As you can see, fat and protein are closely tied together. When most people think about avoiding fat they think about staying away from foods such as the obvious butter and added oils, but they completely forget that many of their favorite foods are full of fat.

Staying away from fat means reducing the amount of protein you eat in a day. The highest fatty foods you probably eat are dairy products; milk and milk products are full of fat (even when they are called slim or low-fat).

You may be worried that if you cut out a lot of animal proteins then you will not be getting enough protein, but the truth is that you are probably getting more than enough protein. The recommended daily allowance from the government suggests that you should be eating somewhere between forty and fifty grams of protein a day (depending on your sex and your body weight). It is currently estimated that most Americans are putting about ninety to one hundred grams of protein in their mouths every day,[19] twice the recommended amount. There is research that suggest that even the government's estimate is too high and that we probably only need around twenty to thirty grams of protein a day.[20]

If you are eating a plant-based diet then you are getting more than enough protein. Beans and nuts are great sources of protein (beans contain twelve to sixteen grams of protein per cup and nuts contain around thirty grams of protein per cup). But even vegetables are a good source of protein, including broccoli (three grams per cup), sweet potatoes (three grams per cup), potatoes (five grams per cup); even carrots, spinach, tomatoes, and onions all contain about one gram of protein per cup.

Getting enough protein is really not a worry when you are eating a balanced diet.

WHICH IS WORSE?

At this point you may be wondering which is worse: eating fat or eating sugars and foods that act like sugars? The answer is that they often work together to spoil your health. Diabetes, in particular, is made much worse by our double dippings of daily sugar and fat.

Imagine what happens inside your body when you eat a high sugar and high-fat meal. Yes, your body might decide to use the fat in the food you are eating as energy, but there is usually no reason to use fat as energy because you are consistently eating throughout the day and throughout your life (whether you are hungry or not). The sugars and other carbohydrates you are constantly consuming more than meet your body's energy needs, so the body has only has one real choice: store that energy as fat. The same is true for all the fat you already have on your body; there is no need to use it when another, easier source of energy is constantly available.

Put yourself in the position of the "energy czar" of your body. It is the czar's job to decide where you get energy to do everything your body needs. Remember that glucose is the preferred energy source for all your body's cells. If a fat molecule or a glucose molecule floats by the energy czar, it will pick the glucose molecule because it requires no energy to send it to the cells of your body (and remember that it also takes almost no energy to store that fat). Using fat for energy only becomes a thought for the energy czar when the easy forms of energy (glucose) are not around.

Take a look at a recent study that shows what happens when people stop eating sugar and foods that act like sugar, but forget to also lower the amount of fat and protein that they are eating. The study, which followed close to a hundred thousand people for twenty years showed that a low-carbohydrate, high-protein diet was associated with an almost doubled risk for cardiovascular disease and cancer than a low-carbohydrate, high vegetable diet.[21]

Yes, you want to eliminate sugars and foods that act like sugars, but you also need to lower your proteins and fat and then eat a lot of fruits and vegetables.

WHAT ABOUT GOOD FATS?

You have probably heard about good fats and that they are important to your health. These fats, called essential fatty acids (EFAs) are called "essential" because you cannot make them in your body and you need to get them in your diet. EFAs (specifically the omega-3 or omega-6 oils) are generally missing from our diets.

As you will see later on, I'm not suggesting that you give up all animal proteins, just dramatically curtail them. An occasional serving of fish will get you the essential fatty acids you need. Adding in raw nuts (walnuts, Brazil nuts, hazelnuts, pecans) to your diet can also be a great source of these essential fats.

Summing it all up

Here is what you want to remember about fats:

- Fats are full of calories (even a small amount of fat is packed with a large number of calories). This means that your waistline increases easier when you eat fats.

- Eating fatty foods raises your cholesterol level. Having a high cholesterol level means you are more likely to have heart disease, cancer, and even hormone-based diseases.

- Trans fats and hydrogenated oils don't belong in your body. Remember that to eliminate these from your diet means avoiding most processed foods.

- Dairy foods are probably your single highest source of bad fats for your body.

- Don't be fooled by white meat, fish, and other proteins; they still contain a large amount of fats even though they are touted as being low fat foods.

- To get enough of the essential fats, eat raw nuts, or the occasional fish.

VEGETABLE MATTERS

You may think that vegetables and fruits are not a key to battling aliens (and losing weight), but they are. This chapter could easily be the shortest in the book; all I would have to write is these five words: eat your vegetables and fruits. But like most advice, vegetable eating is easy to suggest as something we should all do, but most people don't (or won't) do it. Not eating your fruits and veggies is a problem, especially if you have a goal of being healthy and losing weight.

What is it about fruits and vegetables that make them so good for you and, at the same time, so hard to get into your diet? Sure, your mom probably told you over and over again to eat your vegetables, but the only way you were going to eat those green beans was by pinching your nose and forcing yourself to eat the few bites required to allow your escape from the table.

Instead of keeping this chapter super-short, let's take a look at the state of the vegetables and fruits in your diet and see how those sneaky aliens have kept you away from these life-supporting nutrients and what you can do to turn the tables on those aliens and welcome back into your diet the foods your body so desperately needs.

NOT ENOUGH

You don't eat enough fruits and vegetables. How do I know that you don't eat enough fruits and vegetables? It's simple: If you are alive and reading this book then you aren't eating enough fresh fruits and vegetables. Study after study has shown that Americans (and people in most industrialized countries) are not eating enough vegetables.

A report published in the April 2007 issue of the *American Journal of Preventive Medicine* tells us just how bad our fruit and vegetable aversion really is. According to the report, only 11 percent of the population of the United States eats enough fruits and vegetables every day.[22] That sounds bad, but that is just the tip of the iceberg lettuce. "Enough" fruit and vegetables (according to the report) is only two or more fruit servings, or three or more vegetable servings per day (which ain't very much).

But the news gets much worse, because in order to understand how bad these numbers are, you have to understand what they are counting as a fruit and vegetable. Drinking fruit juice is considered a serving of fruit; while pure fruit juice can be considered to be healthy by some, it is not a whole fruit and is missing vital nutrients (most notably, the fiber). Take away fruit juices (especially orange juice) from the counting of servings of fruit and most people in the report weren't eating any fruit at all.

On the vegetable side, the researchers counted potatoes as a vegetable, which would be fine if most of the potatoes were actually potatoes. Other studies show that about forty percent of all the vegetables we eat are potatoes,[23] but most of those are eaten as (you guessed it) French fries.

The aliens love this. Even when we count servings of fruits and vegetables, we are falling into the alien's fiendish plans. A fried fatty vegetable is no vegetable at all and a fruit devoid of fiber (which acts like sugar in the body) that is eaten days after being juiced and shipped across the country is no fruit at all.

If, by this low, low, low standard, only 11 percent of us are eating enough fruits and vegetables and most of the fruits and vegetables that we do eat are highly processed, then it is safe to say that virtually no one in a developed country is eating enough fruits and vegetables (yes, I'm talking about you).

WHY BOTHER?

At this point you might ask the simple question, "Why bother?" What is so great about fruits and vegetables anyway? That is a good question: Fruits and vegetables are not only just good foods to eat, they are the most important food you should be eating because no other type of food on our planet is so high in known (and unknown or undiscovered nutrients) while at the same time being low in calories.

If you just read the previous line and started wondering what an "unknown or undiscovered nutrient" is, let me explain.

Unknown nutrients may be the most important reason you should eat fruits and vegetables. Sure, vegetables and fruits are full of vitamins and minerals and healthy fibers, but that is not the only reason you want to eat more of them. No, you want to eat more fruits and vegetables because they contain other life-thriving nutrients.

The problem stems from our strange perceptions about what foods are and why we eat them. After all, you eat bananas to get more potassium, don't you? We eat oranges for their vitamin C and drink milk to get our calcium. But what comes from this way of looking at food is that we tend to think that vitamins and minerals make up a lot of what we eat when we eat foods, but this is not true.

Foods are full of nutrients that we don't even have proper names for and we are not really sure what they do. If you were to take apart an apple, you might discover that there are about three hundred different chemicals inside that apple. If you were to remove all of the vitamins and minerals from that list, along with the other known nutrients (such as amino and fatty acids) then you would still be left with at least 250 chemicals in a typical apple that our scientists have no idea what they do (let alone have a proper name for).

It is not that human scientists aren't looking for these chemicals; they are. In fact, you have probably heard of about some of the recent discoveries of previously unknown food chemicals such as resveratrol, lycopene, lutein, and others. These non-vitamin nutrients have made recent news for the profound effects they have on our health and longevity (and we are discovering more of these unknown nutrients every day).

Here is the key: potassium pills don't replace our bananas, just as vitamin C doesn't replace our oranges. A banana is much more than just potassium and tomatoes are more than just lycopene. You and human scientists might just as well give up on attributing the health benefits of a certain food to just one nutrient. Foods, it turns out, are more complex than we ever imagined. That apple you ate this morning is providing you with more benefits than we could ever hope to count or quantify. Vegetables and fruits are more than the sum of the nutrients we can measure. There is something in fresh, whole, alive foods for which human (or alien) technology will never account.

We are meant to eat fruits and vegetables; in fact, we are meant to eat a ton of fruits and vegetables. While it might strike you as odd, eating a mostly fruit- and vegetable-based diet is what our bodies were designed to do (and what aliens are happy we don't do). Your sweet tooth has a purpose; it should point you in the direction of fruits (not sugar). Instead of being a side dish, fruits and vegetables should make up the bulk of what goes into our mouths.

Why bother with fruits and vegetables? Because they are the exact foods your body needs to battle disease, keep you healthy, and help you make it through this journey alive.

DISEASE

Let's take a look at what happens when you do something right and increase your consumption of fruits and vegetables:

- Down goes your risk of high blood pressure.[24]
- You also reduce your overall risk of heart disease.[25] Consumption of fruits and vegetables—particularly leafy green vegetables and vitamin C-rich fruits—appears to have a protective effect against coronary heart disease.[26]
- Fruit consumption seems to be protective against cancers of the esophagus, oral cavity, and larynx.
- Eating more fruits and veggies protects against cancer of the stomach and pancreas as well as colorectal, prostate,[27] and bladder cancers. Even lung cancer risk is lower for smokers who eat their veggies.[28]
- For women, cancers of the cervix, ovary, and breast,[29] and endometrium are all lower when they consume more fruits and vegetables.
- The risk for Alzheimer's,[30] diabetes,[31] and many other diseases is lower with higher fruit and vegetable consumption.

Clearly, it is in your best interest to stuff more vegetables and fruits into your diet. But what about weight gain? Vegetables and fruits excel at helping you lose weight. Eating a high plant-based diet is strongly associated with weight loss.[32] There is what is called an "inverse relationship" between the amounts of vegetables and fruits that you eat and your weight; as fruit and vegetable consumption goes up, your weight goes down.[33] In some studies, higher vegetable and fruit consumption means you have a 25 percent less chance of gaining weight.[34] That is huge!

In fact, there is no quicker way to lose weight than to eat only fruits and vegetables (no grains, no meat, no sugars, and no oils) and the great part about that kind of diet plan is that you can eat as much as you want. Let's not jump to such an extreme diet just yet (I'll have much more to say about how to put together a diet plan later in the book), but if you want to munch on apple or some carrots while reading the rest of the book, I strongly support that urge.

FIBER

Since we have been talking about fruits and vegetables and vegetables and fruits, let's take a moment to peer into the subject of fiber.

Earlier we talked about how you had to change what you thought about fat (remember, most of the fat you eat is "hidden" in the protein and dairy foods you consume), but it would also help you to switch the way you think about fiber. When most people think about fiber, they think about a powdery substance that comes in a can or in their oat bran muffins. While those additives certainly are a fiber, the fibers I want you to start thinking about are those found in fruits and vegetables.

Let me stop here and make a small suggestion about your fiber intake: If you have to take a supplement to get enough fiber in your diet, then you are on the wrong path. You can find all the fiber that you need in whole fruits and vegetables.

But what is it about fiber that makes it so great, and how does it fit into your plan to fight aliens and lose weight? The one thing most people know about getting enough fiber is that it keeps you regular (and yes this is true), but what you may not know is that fiber is also one of the main "sweeping" agents of the body. As fiber passes through your digestive tract, it picks up a lot of fat-soluble molecules and other debris and carries them out of your body. This sweeping action is why eating a high-fiber diet lowers cholesterol,[35] but it may also be why there is a lower risk for breast cancer in women who eat a large amount of fiber (fiber takes cholesterol and bad estrogens out of the body).[36]

But the most important reason you want to get enough fiber is that it helps you to lose weight. Here is the secret the aliens don't want you to know: When you eat enough fiber you don't feel as hungry; a belly full of vegetable and fruit fiber is a content and happy belly.

When you eat a high-fat meal that has very little bulk (or fiber) you can still be hungry; the same is true when you drink a soda. You can fill your belly with tons of fat and sugar calories and still think that you need more food. The reason that you don't feel full when you eat these foods is because your belly is empty (it's no wonder that you keep returning to the pantry or the snack machine). The same is not true of high-fiber fruits and vegetables: eat a lot of them and your stomach not only *feels* full, it *is* full.

Feeling full is one thing, but losing weight is another. The question that you are probably wondering is: Does eating a good amount of fiber help you to lose weight? The answer appears to be yes; scientific research has shown that eating more fiber does help to lower your weight.[37]

Do you know what happens to a body designed to eat high-nutrient, low-calorie fruits and vegetables when it is fed low-fiber, high-caloric foods? You get weight gain and you are hungry all the time. Turn that dynamic on its head by finding more fruits and vegetables to sneak into your every meal.

BUT I DON'T LIKE VEGGIES

Okay, we cannot leave the subject of vegetables without discussing the taste issue.

Whenever I mention that vegetables need to be a bigger part of people's diet they almost always tell me that they don't like the taste of vegetables. People have aversions to all sorts of foods, but no other food group receives more turned up noses than the vegetable group. Fruits are something that most people can eat, but suggest that they eat broccoli, kale, green beans, Brussels sprouts, carrots, and other vegetables and they act as if they might die if they had to put these foods in their mouths.

Okay, you got me with this one: most people don't like the taste to vegetables. But let me suggest to you that the reason most people don't like vegetables is that they are eating high fat, high sugar, and highly processed foods, which typically have much stronger tastes that dull your normal taste buds. To understand this, think about someone who drinks straight whisky all the time and what they might think of drinking water (our processed foods are no different than whisky).

While I know you are not going to believe me right now, your tastes do change as you eat less of the high-fat, high sugar, and processed foods. As you adjust to a more whole food diet, your taste buds will come on the journey with you and adapt to your new lifestyle. In fact, you may find that super-sweet, super-salty, and super-fatty foods that you now eat become hard to eat once you avoid them for a while (just as the whisky drinker will find whisky harder to drink after staying away from it for a while).

Take the plunge along with me and start adding more vegetables into your diet and see what a great difference it will make in your life.

Summing it all up

Here is what you want to remember about vegetables:

- Eat your fruits and vegetables

ADDICTIONS

Imagine for a moment how deadly it would be if you were addicted to the very foods that obstruct your health. That, unfortunately, is the exact situation we find ourselves in: the most lethal foods in your diet are also the most addictive. Addictions to foods such as sugar, chocolate, dairy, and even meat are more real than you might have ever imagined.

If you look at what we are eating through the lens of addictions, you notice that we jump from addicting food to addicting food throughout the whole day, trying desperately to hold our mood and energy in balance.

If you are a typical person, you start your day with either a caffeinated beverage (tea, coffee) or something sweet (or both). That sugar and caffeine rush will last you a few hours until you start to feel tired later in the day. Your fatigue and sluggish mind then drive you to find another cup of coffee or something sweet (or both). You bounce from highs to lows throughout the day until you arrive home at the end of the day, frazzled or stressed out (or both). It is no wonder you reach for something alcoholic (beer, wine, hard alcohol) or calming like ice cream (or both) to take that edge off.

If you eat something that makes you feel tired or down then you look for that stimulant to bring you back up. Have you ever eaten a large amount of fried foods and then found yourself desperately needing something sweet to balance it out? Or have you ever overdosed on potato chips (or some other snack) and knew you needed coffee or you wouldn't make it through the rest of the day? These are our self-medicating routines. It is as if we all are trying to maintain a happy and energized state all the time and when we fall out of that balance it is time to reach for some sort of fix. This all reminds me (once again) of rats in a cage. If they have free access to heroin, at first they only use the drug occasionally but as time goes by they use all the time.

While we like to think that we are in control of what we eat, the addictive substances inside of these foods sing sweet Siren songs to our brains, seducing and enticing us throughout the day to continue to put them in our mouths. Scientists are just beginning to understand how powerful these addictions are. Let's take a look at one of the best known of these addictions: sugar.

SUGAR BRAINS

For years people have been saying (half-jokingly) that they are addicted to sugar, but no one seriously considered sugar to be a real addiction. That all changed when scientists started looking closer at the brains of people and animals when they ate sugar and compared those sugar-high brains to brains addicted to other substances like cigarettes, alcohol, and even hard drugs. The big surprise to everyone was that there is almost no difference between a brain addicted to sugar and a brain addicted to those other substances.

While studying human brains is possible, most of the research on sugar addiction has been done on rats. Let's peek in on researchers who have decided to see what happens when they let rats eat all the sugar they want.

- If you give rats free access to as much sugar as they want, they will eat it more than any other food in their cage. Many rats will eat *only* sugar, to the point that they become very ill.[38]
- If you addict a rat to sugar and then take sugar away from them, the rats tremble, shake, become anxious, their teeth chatter, and they become more aggressive. These are the exact symptoms you get when you addict rats to other drugs such as nicotine, alcohol, or morphine.[39] These behaviors, by the way, are all the classic signs of withdrawal.
- If you addict a rat to sugar, take it away from them for a period of time, and then let them have sugar back again, they will gorge themselves. Does this sound anything like the last diet you were on? You were able to stay on the diet until you ate something forbidden and then it was all over. This is another hallmark sign of addiction: removal and return of the addiction always causes binging.[40]

- When put under stress, rats eat more sugar.[41]
- The brains of rats addicted to sugar are almost identical to the brains of rats addicted to alcohol, nicotine, or other hard drugs. Sugar actually causes physical changes to the brain similar to other addictions.[42]
- The most remarkable studies are those when scientists addict rats to sugar and then give them a drug called an opioid antagonist. Giving opioid antagonists to a rat addicted to drugs like morphine or nicotine produces withdrawal symptoms. The same is true for sugar. Give an opioid antagonist to a sugar-addicted rat and they will tremble, pace the cage, their teeth will chatter, and they will become aggressive, proving how similar sugar addiction is to other drug addictions.[43]

Being addicted to sugar isn't just something to joke about when you can't resist the candy machine or that piece of birthday cake. Sugar addiction means that you don't have as much control as you thought you did over what goes into your mouth. It means you are eating when you are not even hungry. It means that you might try a diet and be fine until you put something sweet into your mouth and then you are on a binge and you gain back all the weight you lost. It means you are going to have a very hard time changing your diet (and the aliens know this), but sugar addiction is far from the end of our addiction story.

MORE ADDICTIONS

Sugar is not the only addiction we face. Research has shown that our mouths love the taste of fatty and salty foods,[44] and this too might well be considered an addiction. Food addictions are the subject of a well-researched book called *Breaking the Food Seduction,* by Neal Barnard, MD. You should pick this book up and read it, but let me give you the highlights about food addictions according to Dr. Barnard:

- **Dairy foods**: Milk, cheese, yogurt, and other milk products all contain casomorphins.[45] Morphine, as you may know, is a highly addictive substance and is found in our milk in the form of a casomorphine (a milk morphine). Why does milk have morphine in it? It helps to ensure that babies enjoy breastfeeding. Morphine is also calming and may be the reason you reach for ice cream or milk at the end of a long stressed-out day.
- **Caffeine**: The addictive qualities of caffeine are well known and I won't belabor them here, but know that many foods besides coffee and tea contain caffeine (including chocolate).
- **Chocolate**: Chocolate contains many addictive substances (no wonder we all need our chocolate fix). Chocolate contains sugar, caffeine, and theobromine (substances known as methylxanthines) that encourage our addiction.[46] Chocolate even contains marijuana-like substances.[47]
- **Meat**: There is some evidence that even meats contain addictive substances.

Addictions are nothing to joke about and they have a serious impact on your health and your waistline. Addictions are why you often eat more than you should; they also partly responsible for that whole bag of chips you ate last week (even when you were not hungry). Addictions, more than anything, are probably what cause you to bounce back to the same (or even higher) weight than before you started on a diet plan.[48] Food addictions are the key to understanding what keeps pulling you back into your old habits when you want to move forward. There are other addictive substances in our food stream, but I'll leave it to you to pick up Dr. Barnard's book if you want to learn more.

ADDICTION ADDITION

The key to understanding addictions is to know that they all work together. Addictions are bad enough on their own but they also tend to attract other addictive substances. If you are using one addictive substance then you are likely to use another. While this thinking is kind of like the "gateway" theory of drug abuse, it does appear to be true. Drinking alcohol leads to more smoking and many people report that caffeine increases their desire for sugary foods. Sugar, in turn, increases the desire for salty foods, and so on....

Does this mean that you have to quit all addictive substance all at once? Probably not, but you do have to pay attention to how these addictions tend to feed one another. If something you are doing makes it hard to stick to your dietary plans then think about removing it.

WHY BRING UP ADDICTIONS?

At this point in the book you may be throwing up your hands wondering how you will ever get out of eating the foods that you now eat and get on to a path of health and wellness. I bring up addictions not to depress you but to let you know two things:

- **First**: Addictions are real and hard to get over. If you want to remove sugar, salt, fat, or other foods from your life, you should prepare for a battle.
- **Second**: It does get better. You may fall down a bit, but it will get better.

Let me tell you that you have no idea how bad you feel right now until you have given up addictive foods and set yourself on a healthier course. When you clean up your diet, you are going to feel great and have a lot of energy. That weight you have been carrying around is going to take a permanent vacation from your body when you adjust your foods to what your body needs.

Take it easy with yourself as you work through this program and your addictions. Some things you are going to find easy; others are going to be a struggle. You might find it all easy at first and then have it fall apart later on. Pick yourself up and start again; you and your life are worth the effort.

Summing it all up

Here is what you want to remember about addictions:

- You have addictions and it is going to be hard to kick them.
- Things get better (much better) when you are eating real foods.

HAVE ALIENS STOLEN MY METABOLISM?

This chapter is the icing on the cake (at least for the aliens) and it will answer the puzzle about where you metabolism disappeared to and what you can do about finding it again. This chapter is going to be a bit more involved than the rest because your metabolism is a tricky landscape; it takes a while to navigate through our metabolic jungle. But fear not, my intrepid explorer: I will show you just how your metabolism was stolen and, more importantly, how you can get it back. Exploring what has gone wrong with your metabolism is a key to understanding why the rest of the alien's plan to make you overweight and oversick works so well.

Every recipe needs cooking instructions, and the alien recipe for making fat and sick humans is no different. Aliens, however, don't use an oven to make humans sick; they use your inactivity. This is because being inactive makes everything else that you are doing (eating sugar, fat, salt, no vegetables) much worse and destroys your metabolism. If you are searching for your lost metabolism, then I have some good news and some bad news for you. The good news is that your metabolism is recoverable; the bad news is that it is going to take some work on your part to get it back.

What is the connection between your inactivity and your metabolism? Well, I'm glad you asked because it is important to your health; let's take a look.

WHERE DID MY METABOLISM GO?

If you could go back in time and watch your life as an outsider, there are a few things you might notice about the changes to your metabolism over your lifetime.

The first thing you might notice is that the change to your metabolism didn't happen all that fast (at least at first). Most people gain a pound or two and then hold a steady weight for a while (for months or even years), then they gain a few more pounds. This pattern may go on for a long time and then (just like a switch being thrown) they gain a bunch of weight in a short period of time. This last stage is what gives the impression that your metabolism failed all at once, when, in fact, it had been changing for a long time.

The second thing you would notice by watching your metabolism over time is that your activity level has probably decreased since you were a child. It is no surprise that your activity level has dropped because every extra pound of weight you put on makes exercise only that much more difficult.

Over the years you may have even tried to lose weight and had some success, but then the pounds you lost just jumped right back on. This, you will find out, is a trick of your metabolism: If you reduce the number of calories you are eating, your metabolism slows down. It is tough to win the weight war when your metabolism is working against you. Research shows that people can typically lose about 10 percent of their body weight, but then they yo-yo back up to their previous weight again. The culprit responsible for that yo-yo effect is your metabolism (and aliens).

To understand how your metabolism has turned against you, you first have to understand what a "feed-forward" cycle is. A feed-forward cycle is a mechanism during which creating something makes it easier to create more of that something (sort of like having money makes it easier to make more money). In your body, these feed-forward cycles can work for you or against you.

Your metabolism is a good example of a feed-forward cycle. In your body it works like this: gaining weight means it is easier to gain more weight. The problem is that this is the feed-forward cycle you are working against all the way down to your ideal weight. You have to fight your body's tendency to put on more weight; while it is not impossible, it is going to be a fight.

Most people think that their metabolism is a one-way street: Once your metabolism has slowed there is no way to get it back. This is not true. The worst thing you can do is throw your hands up in the air in disgust and give up the fight, because that is when your metabolism really starts to work against you. Your metabolism may have taken some time off, but it is out there just waiting for you to give it a jumpstart again and then, instead of being a hated enemy, your metabolism will once again be on your side.

WHAT IS METABOLISM?

Metabolism is kind of a funny concept and we should talk about exactly what it is before moving on.

Metabolism can be described as all the chemical reactions that take place in our bodies throughout a day. In metabolism, some substances are broken down to create energy (catabolism), while other substances are built up and created (anabolism). Total body metabolism accounts for both the digestion of food and the total amount of energy used in the body. But even that doesn't really mean anything, does it?

What you need to know about metabolism is that everything that happens in your body is some sort of chemical reaction and that each of these chemical reactions takes some amount of energy. So, for our purposes, let's consider metabolism to be *the total amount of energy that we burn in a day*. We have many ways of measuring how much energy our bodies use in a day but the most useful for us is something called the **Basal Metabolic Rate** or BMR. We are going to talk a lot about your BMR. It can be your best friend or worst enemy when it comes to weight loss.

BMR is a measurement that scientists calculate to tell them just how much energy your body uses in a day. What is important about BMR is that it is a measurement of the amount of energy you use even if you were just laying in a bed, doing nothing, all day long. Your BMR is a measurement of all the processes that go on in your body: from operating your brain, to beating your heart, to processing waste, to moving blood around, and everything else your body does to keep you alive. BMR accounts for all the energy you need to run your body, but it does not include anything you do once you are out of bed and walking around.

That means that doing the dishes, walking, having sex, cleaning up the house, playing, sneezing, or running in a marathon are all NOT included in the BMR.

Here is the key reason BMR is important and your best friend in weight loss: Your BMR uses more energy than almost anything you can do all day long. Read that again: *Your Basal Metabolic Rate burns more energy than anything else you do.*

To give you an idea about how much energy your BMR burns, imagine that there was a competition between you and your BMR to see who used more calories in a day. Put on your running shoes, step out the door, and start running; guess how long would you have to run to match the amount of calories burned by your BMR in a typical day? In truth, this is a difficult calculation, but for the average person running at moderate speeds (12 mph) it would take around three to four hours of constant running to match the amount of energy your BMR burns every day.

I don't know about you, but I don't have time to run four hours every day (nor do I really want to try); this is why your BMR is the king calorie burner in your body. Remember, your Basal Metabolic Rate is the amount of calories you burn each day even if you were to never move from your bed. The average, healthy adult's BMR is burning around 1200 to 1800 calories a day (or somewhere between 50 and 75 percent of your daily caloric expenditure).

The way I figure it, you have two choices when you want to burn more calories: You can either spend several hours running every day or you can learn how to increase your Basal Metabolic Rate. Exercise and BMR are actually closely related, but before we get to that, we need to look closer at our energy expenditure.

ENERGY EXPENDITURE

I mentioned earlier that your Basal Metabolic Rate is made up of all the energy processes going on in your body, but there are different parts of your body that use more energy than others (all body parts are not created equally).

Take a look at this chart and see where your energy is being spent:

BMR Energy Expenditure	
Liver	27 %
Brain	19 %
Heart	7 %
Kidneys	10 %
Muscle	18 %
Other organs	19 %

You can see from the chart that different parts of your body need more energy than others. If you look closely you will notice that one of the items on the chart is different than all the others. Do you see it? The difference is important because it is the only item on the chart that you are able to change. Take another look: Did you see it this time?

Some people say that they can change their heart function, and that is true. Other people say that they can increase the amount of thinking that they do and they are correct there too (using your brain doesn't change the amount of energy the brain uses—at least not enough to make a difference in weight loss).

The only part of your BMR that you can change is your muscle mass. You can't really change the function or functioning of any of your organs, but you do have control over the amount of muscle mass you have on your body. There is the simple answer you were looking for: If you want to increase you BMR, you have to increase your muscle mass. More muscle in your body means higher BMR and higher BMR means more calorie burning all day (and night) long.

Actually, let's look a little closer at what can change your metabolism.

METABOLISM MODIFIERS

Your metabolism is far from being static and unchangeable; there are a lot of things that can alter your metabolism.

- **Age:** I hate to tell you this, but your metabolism slows as you age. But the typical slowing of your metabolism as you age may not be as inevitable as it seems. Yes, most people's metabolism does slow as they age but that doesn't mean that it is normal (remember that there is a big difference between what appears to be normal and what is normal— the "rats in a cage" syndrome) Most people also tend to decrease muscle mass and increase body fat as they age and this leads to lower metabolism (see below).
- **Body Size:** The taller and thinner you are, the higher your BMR.
- **Body Composition:** The more muscle mass you have and the lower your body fat, the higher your BMR. This is because muscle is metabolically active tissue (it burns a lot of calories).
- **Low Calorie Diet:** Eating a low-calorie diet actually *decreases* BMR. A severely restricted diet can reduce your metabolic rate by as much as 30 percent. Remember this: low calories leads to low metabolism, so forget starvation diets.
- **Breast Feeding and Pregnancy:** Both breast-feeding and pregnancy increase BMR. This is not much help for most of us, but good to know.
- **Exercise:** Exercise can increase BMR for up to forty-eight hours. Read that again: specific types of exercise can increase BMR for up to two days!
- **Sex:** Unfair, but true: BMR is higher in males than in females even at the same body weight; this has to do with the amount of muscle mass men carry compared to women, and female hormones tend to add fat more easily than male hormones.
- **Stress:** BMR is higher in times of emotional stress. We all know people who have lost weight after someone close to them died or other some other tragic life event. You might be thinking you could put yourself under emotional stress

just to increase your BMR, but this kind of diet plan would have horrible effects on the rest of your body and is not worth trying.

• **Weather:** BMR is higher in both cold and very hot weather.

LOW CALORIES MEANS MORE WEIGHT

I have to mention this again because it is so important: Dramatically reducing your calories does two things that actually make it harder to lose weight.

The first is that it tells your body that you are in starvation mode. Your body will take this as a sign to make sure it stores as much fat as possible. Every morsel of food you put in your mouth is guaranteed to be stored as fat because your body thinks you are not getting enough calories.

We have also discussed how low-calorie diets can cause up to a 30 percent drop in metabolism; muscles are one of the reasons for this drop. As you starve yourself not only are more food calories turned into fat because your body thinks it will never see another calorie again, but your body also steals calories from itself. While you might think this is a good idea, it's not. Your body turns to muscles to supply your energy needs just as much as it turns to fat, so when you go on a low-calorie diet, you are losing muscle *and* fat (not a good combination).

Losing muscle means that you are lowering your BMR. This is especially true if you are on a low-calorie diet and not exercising. You might think that you can get away with eating a low-calorie diet and exercising to keep your muscles, but even this doesn't work very long; you will still lose muscle mass. The key to good weight loss is to provide the muscles with what they need by eating enough good quality foods and then increase the total amount of muscle mass by proper exercising.

When you are restricting calories, you are also robbing your brain of the basic building blocks of brain chemicals that make you feel satisfied and full. No wonder you are hungry all the time when you go on a low-calorie diet.

What is the take-home message from all of this? Don't hang all your weight-loss hopes on the amount of calories you put in your body versus how many calories you burn. It is much more important to change *what* you put in your mouth than *how much.*

INCREASING YOUR METABOLISM

After reading the previous pages, you will notice that there are many things that can change your metabolism in good or bad ways, but only a few over which you really have control. Since we can't do anything about how old we are, or whether we are male or female, let's look at what we can change.

MUSCLES

As you may have guessed by reading this far, muscles are the first key to increasing your Basal Metabolic Rate. Muscles account for around 20 percent of your total BMR; the more muscles you have the more calories you burn every day and night just sitting there doing nothing. For every pound of muscle you have, you are burning around 50 calories a day.

Muscles are a two-for-one deal, because not only are they more metabolically active (burn more calories) than most other tissue in the body when you are not moving around, they also burn more energy when you *are* moving around. So, every time you exercise, clean the house, walk to your car, or go shopping, you are burning even more calories.

The good news doesn't stop there. Whenever you participate in some sort of muscle-building activity, such as lifting weights, you have just kicked your metabolism into high gear for the next forty-eight hours. By some estimates, that extra "kick" amounts to a 10 percent increase in your BMR.[49,50] For most people, this is 100 to 200 more calories burned every day just sitting still doing nothing. While that 100 calories might not sound like much, that it is an extra 3000 to 6000 calories a month that don't end up on your hips and all you have to do is exercise every day or every other day to keep your metabolism revved up.

Before we move on, let's do the math on the calorie-burning potential of more muscle mass. Let's say that you worked out for a few months and added five pounds of muscles to your body and that you are exercising every other day. What would that do for you?

That extra five pounds of muscles will be burning 250 calories a day (each pound of muscle burns 50 calories a day). Now that you have that extra muscle you will be burning more calories with everything that you do; let's say that amounts to an extra 100 calories a day (it could be more if you are more active). Since you are now exercising every other day, you get the metabolic kick of an extra 100 to 200 calories burning off every day. Let's not forget the calories burned from the exercise itself—add in another 100 calories a day (this is a low estimate and takes in to account you are only exercising every other day). What do you get for your effort? Here is a chart that sums it all up:

	Day	Month
Extra muscle	250 calories	7,500 calories
Activity	100 calories	3,000 calories
Metabolism	100 calories	3,000 calories
Exercise	100 calories	3,000 calories
TOTAL:	550 calories	16,500 calories

What you get from all of your effort is a calorie-burning machine. Remember that one pound of fat is equal to 3500 calories and that the estimates above are all conservative (you could be burning much more). If you have followed the above plan, you are burning an extra five pounds of body fat every month (that's sixty pounds in a year). What you also have to remember is that we are only talking about exercise here; if you add in the rest of the fight against the alien's diet plan, you weight loss will be outstanding.

CHANGE YOUR MIND ABOUT EXERCISE

We have been thinking about exercise all wrong. When you read that one pound of fat contains 3,500 calories and walking fast for a mile will only burn off around 100 calories, who wouldn't get discouraged? Here is what you need to wrap your mind around about exercise: You don't exercise to burn off calories; you exercise to boost your metabolism so that your BMR will burn more calories.

The next question that comes to mind is "What kind of exercises should you do?"

Metabolism-boosting exercises come in two flavors: aerobic exercise (exercise that gets your heart racing) and muscle-building exercise. Both weight lifting and aerobic exercise can increase your metabolism. Simply doing anything that gets you up and moving around builds muscles. The muscles you want to build in your body are the large muscles of your legs and arms. Walking, running, biking, golf, swimming, bowling, tennis, and a variety of other sports will add to your muscle mass. But if you really want to build muscle, you have to consider doing some kind of weight training.

The types of exercise you need to do need to be fairly intense in order to boost your metabolism, but you can make changes slowly and build over time. Most people find they enjoy their new bodies and their new lives much more when they start exercising. I'll have more to say about weight lifting and specifically how intense your exercise must be when we get specific about how to put together your own personal plan.

Summing it all up

Here is what you want to remember about your Metabolism:

- You lost your metabolism, but you can get it back.
- Your Basal Metabolic Rate (BMR) burns more calories than anything else you can do.
- Muscles make up the biggest part of the BMR that you can change.
- You have to exercise to change your BMR.

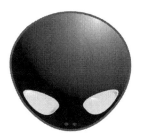

FIGHT THE ALIENS' DIET PLAN

I don't know if you can hear what I hear, but stop what you are doing right now and go to a quiet place. If you take a moment and listen very closely, you can hear the agonizing scream of someone clutching their chest and writhing in pain. Before this person even has time to hit the ground, another agonizing scream reaches your ears.

What is the sound you are hearing? That is the sound of someone having a heart attack; it happens every twenty seconds of every day of every week of the year. In case you think that sound is coming only from men, it is not. Almost one half of all heart attacks occur in women and heart attacks are much more deadly in women (a larger percentage of women are dead a year after their first heart attack than men).

I mentioned earlier that you do not have the luxury of separating your health from your weight loss; they are one and the same. You can try to trick your body by going on a crazy diet or taking some mad scientist's magic pill. You might lose some pounds, but you are still on your way to joining the choir of people who are paying the price for a diet designed by aliens.

You are, in a very real sense, standing at a crossroads.

If you are like most of us, you have been eating food that is tasty for your tongue but alien to your body. You are at this crossroads because if you continue to eat this way, you are going to live a life like everyone around you. While that might not seem like a bad thing, let me tell you what is happening to everyone around you.

You, of course, don't need me to tell you that things are bad. The morning I wrote this, I noticed an article that says, once again, that Americans are getting fatter. The article reports that Colorado has the lowest rate of obesity in the United States (with only 21.8 percent of my home state's population considered obese). While that sounds great for Colorado, it isn't, especially when you look at how things have changed over time. The same study reported that in 1991 there was *no* state that had over 20 percent of their population considered obese. Think about that: the skinniest state today would have been the fattest twenty years ago.

But let's stop talking about the general population and start talking about you. Take a moment to think about your future. What do you see? If you are like most people, here is what you expect out of your life:

When you are young, you are full of energy and excitement about life. You go on adventures, try new things. But as you age (maybe in your forties or even in your thirties) your doctor is going to suggest that you start taking your first prescription. Maybe your first drug is for high cholesterol, or maybe it is for high blood pressure, or maybe it is for blood sugar control. You are now also gaining weight and exercising less because you are too busy with the everyday demands of your life. As you age, you are thinking about getting diseases such as diabetes, heart disease, cancer, arthritis, or Alzheimer's.

Isn't that what you are expecting out of your life? While you might not think you are expecting a future like that, you are, because that is what you see all around you every day. You probably don't know anyone who has escaped heart disease, cancer, or diabetes as they have aged. But here is the crazy thing: You don't have to die of one of those diseases; researchers suggest that as many as 75 percent of diabetes, heart disease, and cancer are preventable.

You are at a crossroads and your health is in your hands.

You can either choose to do what all your neighbors are doing and suffer the same fate as them, or you can turn your life around and start eating what humans are supposed to eat. Even if you have started medications and have diabetes or heart disease, there is still a chance you can reverse your disease. How do I know? Because people who have refused to live in the rat's cage anymore are making changes to the way that they are living and what they are eating and they are losing weight and feeling better.

Your future is in your hands. You have to make a conscious decision to stop being a rat in a cage. Should you choose to change, you will have a battle ahead of you, not only with yourself: many of your friends, family, and coworkers (not to mention your daily dose of advertising) may resist your change. Will you fall down and make mistakes? Probably. But that doesn't mean you have to stop trying; there is plenty of help out there.

The rest of this book is about making those changes, so let's get going.

WHERE ARE YOU GOING?

First, let me tell you where you are going.

You want 90 percent of everything that goes into your mouth to be a vegetable, fruit, or bean.

What this goal means is that you eat fruits, beans, and vegetables 90 percent of the time. You can eat meat or grains the rest of the time. This (in case you don't know) is an outlandish goal, but it is the only real way you are going to escape the rat cage in which you are living. On top of what you are eating, I'm going to ask you to also exercise. While it might sound to you that you are far away from these goals, you are actually much closer than you think. I'm going to break this program up into easily digestible pieces that help you to discover what parts of the program work for you.

When you are eating mostly fruits and vegetables, you are setting yourself aside from most of the humans around you and you are setting yourself on a course to not only reach your perfect weight, but also to improve your health and live a longer and happier life.

The question you might have at this point is: How can you make the switch from what you are eating right now to what you should be eating? I could give you a list of all the vegetables, beans, and fruits you should be eating and leave it at that, but you deserve something much better.

I've devised a series of experiments for you to try. Each of these experiments last for only a week and will focus you on a certain aspect of your health. I did this so that you can learn how to make the change from where you are to a much healthier place.

EXPERIMENTS

Each of the experiments on the following pages focuses on a different aspect of your weight gain. The way they work is to have you avoid or eat more of a certain kind of food for a week (or more) and see what it does for your weight loss.

Why experiments? Because health takes practice. If you are going to change from what you are eating right now to eating the way your body wants you to, you are going to have to learn new skills. The skills that help you most are those that you teach yourself, not what I (or anyone else) tell you. Take the experiments as just that: experiments. It is a time to try new things, stretch yourself, and learn from your experimenting. You need to practice becoming healthier and making new choices and this takes time.

The problem with most diets is that when you fail to follow them perfectly, you feel like are off the diet and go back to your old ways. Changing your diet by doing experiments means you can try keeping something like sugar out of your diet for a week and then take what you have learned from that experiment and move on to the next experiment. Maybe after your first sugar experiment you find that you still put some sugar in your coffee, but have decided to never drink a soda again. That is great progress! Maybe the next time you choose to try that same sugar-free experiment, you realize that you don't need that sugar in your coffee after all.

The experiment approach gives you the chance to succeed and fail without ever really failing. You get better at whatever you practice; every time you try to kick sugar (or fat, or add in more vegetables…) you learn tricks to keep you on track to a healthier and skinner you.

I can tell you right now that if you were to try all the experiments at once, you would be shocked at how much weight you would lose in a short amount of time. This is because you would be eating exactly what your body was designed to eat, but there are many ways to try these experiments; pick the one that works for you.

PICK ONE

So how do you approach these experiments? It is really up to you. Let me give you a few options and then tell you which one is my favorite.

- The first option is to **try each of the experiments for a week** and see how they work for you. When you are done with the first experiment, stop doing it and move on to the next one.
- You can also **try the each of the experiments for thirty days (instead of a week) at a time**. This one is good because it addresses what I call a "habit barrier." This barrier is typically about three weeks long and is the time that it takes to create a new habit in your life. While you can try any of these experiments for any amount of time you want, think about this one if you are really looking to change your habits.
- You can also **add a new experiment every week**. Here you choose one experiment a week and then add the next one

(while still doing the ones you have already started) for a total of six weeks.

- The last way to try the experiments is to dive in and do them **all at the same time**. This is perhaps the hardest way to approach the experiments, but can also be the easiest. Dramatic changes are sometimes easier than making slow change over time.

The approach that works for most people is to try each of the experiments for a week and then add in the next experiment while continuing the previous experiments. This means you are making changes every week, but not too many at one time. I have arranged the experiments in an order that gives you the most bang for your buck (meaning you will lose the most weight by following them in the order that I've given you). There are a total of six experiments (six weeks to complete them all). You will find that some of the experiments overlap a bit, so they get easier as you go along.

BEFORE YOU START

In the following description of the experiments, I'm going to assume that you are going to try a new experiment every week while keeping the other experiments going. If you decide on a different way of doing the experiments that is fine.

Take a look at all the experiments and notice that there are some you will probably find easier than others because you naturally already take steps toward those. While getting through all the experiments may look daunting at first, you are already closer than you think. As with any experiment, you may fail at times. I would suggest that you try to do the best that you can (but try not to be hard on yourself if you fail; they are experiments, after all). The key here is to learn strategies that will help you get closer to a goal of eating a 90 percent plant-based diet and exercising. Before you get going, I would suggest that you read the chapter on the road less traveled for tips and tricks on how to get through the program.

> ### *Warning!*
>
> If you are taking prescription drugs (especially drugs that change your blood sugar) talk with your doctor before starting any of these experiments. When you avoid all sugars and foods that act like sugars, increase the amount of vegetables you are eating, and start exercising I can guarantee you that your blood sugar will change. If you are taking medications for blood sugar control, you might find yourself with dangerously low blood sugar (which can be life threatening). The same holds true for many other medications; when in doubt, contact your doctor or other health provider.
>
> I strongly encourage everyone to work with their doctor or health care provider whenever they are going to make any dietary change.

EXPERIMENT NUMBER 1: EXERCISE

Exercise is the best place to start any weight loss program. While it might not be *where* you want to start a weight loss program, it is still the best place to start. Remember that exercise improves not only your weight loss, but many other conditions (such as depression, anxiety, sleep, heart disease, diabetes, etc.). You should come to view exercise to be as essential as breathing and drinking water; you cannot survive without it.

More importantly (for you and your weight-loss goals), exercise is the best tool you have to change your metabolism. Remember if you want your metabolism to change you are going to have to get up off your butt and move it around at bit. If you have tried to exercise before and not lost weight, the reason may have been that you weren't exercising in the correct manner or for long enough. You already had to read a long chapter on how your metabolism works and I won't bore you with the technical aspects of just how you should be exercising for weight loss. I created a section in the back of the book (in appendix A), take a look anytime you feel that you are ready to step up your exercise plan. For now, though, you can start exercising, building muscle, and changing your metabolism by choosing almost any exercise.

For some of you who are reading this book, exercise is as foreign as the space aliens using us as experiments; just walking to your mailbox may be a chore. If this is you, start where you can and set small goals to push yourself a little harder every day. If your joints cause you pain, then you can exercise in the water or on an exercise bike; the important thing here is to just pick something and do it.

HOW TO EXERCISE

Okay, here is your exercise plan. You have to use your butt muscles for something other than a seat cushion. For this first experiment, you need to commit to exercising at least twenty minutes every day for the next seven days.

Any exercise you can do (including just walking to the end of the block) will help. Consider starting where you are and pushing yourself a little bit more every day. Think about an exercise you enjoyed as a child and do that. Try biking, walking, running, swimming, or dancing; get a video or DVD, get a friend, take a pet, take a class… just find something to get your heart rate up and commit to it for seven days.

People who like the technical stuff or people who already exercise regularly can skip ahead to Appendix A and learn about what scientists are saying about how hard and how long we need to exercise in order to really supercharge our weight loss.

TRICKS OF THE TRADE

There are a lot of tricks that can help you get started and keep going with your exercise program; you can read my favorites below. If you have any tricks that you like, make sure you stop by www.thealiendiet.com and share them with the rest of us.

I like to incorporate exercise into my day. If I need to go to the store to get groceries, I ride my bike. If I need stamps, I take a walk. Not everyone can do this, but you would be surprised what is within walking or biking distance from your house.

I also suggest that people "pay" for the television they watch by putting some form of exercise equipment (a stationary bike, and elliptical trainer…) in front of the TV. Make a rule for yourself that you cannot watch your shows at night unless you have "paid" for the right to sit there by exercising (you can even do both at the same time).

Remember from the chapter on metabolism that your whole goal with exercise is not to burn calories (although that is nice); your goal is to increase the amount of muscle mass you have (and that will take time). Any exercise that uses the large muscles of the legs and arms will help you to build more muscle and start changing your metabolism.

You may come home at the end of the day thinking that there is no way you can exercise because you are so tired. What you will learn if you start an exercise program is that exercise actually gives you more energy.

If you are having difficulty just getting started, try this trick: tell yourself that you are only going to exercise for five minutes and then you will stop if you don't feel like it. I find that the biggest resistance I have to exercise is just getting started; once I'm out running and my heart is pumping I start enjoying what I'm doing and forget all about my five-minute agreement.

Remember to check with your doctor before starting any exercise program, especially if you have a health condition or you are on medications. Once again, for diabetics, exercise can change the amount of medications you need and you should check in with your health care provider before beginning any exercise program.

EXPERIMENT NUMBER 2: KICK THE SUGAR

Okay, you made it through your first week and have started exercising. Great job! Why don't you make a commitment right now to keep the exercise up for the entire six weeks? If you are really crazy, why don't you commit to exercising for the rest of your life? Sure, there will be times when you don't exercise because of illness, or weather, or some other life event; just plan on those times happening and then starting your exercise program again when things get back to normal. You body and your scale will love you for it.

Let's take a look at your next step: Kicking sugar out of your life. For this week, I want you to focus on kicking all of those extra or added sugars out of your life (we'll talk about the foods that act like sugars next week). So, what does it mean to kick added sugars out of your life? Here is the list of the sweeteners and sugars that can sneak their way into your food:

Agave	Invert sugar
Beet sugar	Lactose
Brown sugar	Malt
Cane sugar	Maltitol
Concentrated grape juice	Maltodextrin
Confectioner's sugar	Maltose
Corn sweeteners	Mannitol
Corn syrup	Maple syrup
Crystallized cane juice	Molasses
Dextrin	Powdered sugar
Dextrose	Rapadura
Evaporated cane juice	Raw sugar
Fructose	Sorbitol
Fruit juice concentrate	Sorghum
Galactose	Sucrose
Glucose	Table sugar
High-fructose corn syrup	Turbinado sugar
Honey	White sugar

Many people think that natural sugars such as turbinado sugar, raw cane sugar, agave, honey, maple syrup, and others are better for you, but they are not. These sugars act the same as every other sugar once they reach your bloodstream. They may seem natural, but they are not; every one of those sugars is concentrated and processed and not found in nature (except for honey – which is processed by bees).

Remember that artificial sweeteners are no good either; keep them out of your diet. They only keep you craving sugars and may even cause you to increase the number of calories you eat in a day.

If you simply have to have something sweet, eat fruit. Fruits contain sugars but you shouldn't worry about the sugars that are naturally occurring in fruit (unless you eat a lot of them). While farmers have bred many fruits to contain more sugars (take a look at the history of apples), they generally have little impact on your blood sugar because fruits also contain a large amount of fiber, which slows down the absorption of sugars in to your bloodstream.

DON'T FREAK OUT

For this week, you are going to find yourself looking at a lot of labels and discovering that almost everything you eat contains some form of sugar in it. All this label reading might drive you a bit crazy. There is a point, though, when you should stop obsessing over what is on the label. You can find peanut butter, salad dressing, and other foods without sugar and you should make the switch to these low-sugar foods, but if you are reading the ingredients on labels and one of the above sugars is very low on the list (ingredients are listed by the amount found in the food) then I wouldn't worry too much about it.

You can't completely avoid all sugar in your diet (even if you wanted to) and you do need some forms of carbohydrates in your diet. I have put many people on a sugar-free diet and some people write me and say that they can't find anything to eat because when they look at labels almost every food contains carbohydrates (and this is true). Don't focus on the amount of carbohydrate in a food; just look to see if added sugar is one of the foods high on the list of ingredients. When in doubt, your tongue will let you know.

WHAT TO EXPECT

Kicking sugar, more than the other experiments, may cause you problems. Remember, you are trying to stop a serious addiction and you might experience withdrawal symptoms. Read the section later in the book about **What to Expect from the Ride** that will help you deal with withdrawal symptoms.

The goal for this week is to stay away from all forms of added sugar to the best of your ability. You will find it easier after the first few days when your taste buds readjust to your new lifestyle and the energy you thought was lost forever comes back.

EXPERIMENT NUMBER 3: FOODS THAT ACT LIKE SUGARS

Okay, you made it through two weeks; here is your week three experiment: Stay away from the foods that act like sugars. As you might remember there are many foods that act like sugars in your body. When you eat these foods you might as well be eating white sugar because these foods (mostly grains) cause your blood sugar to raise the same as if you were eating table sugar. While most people find it fairly easy to stay away from added sugar, staying away from the foods that act like sugars can be a bit more difficult.

The foods that act like sugars fall into two categories: highly processed foods and processed grains. Potato chips, corn chips (chips in general), French fries, donuts, bagels, bread, fruit rollups, and other processed foods should all be kept off your plate, as well as all grains. The biggest sources of foods that act like sugars in your diet are the grains. This means that during this week you stay away from all grains and all foods made from grains. Some grains are good for you when you eat them as a whole grain, but most of the time we eat grains they are just sugar foods. Yes, alcohol is in this group as well and should be avoided.

Processing is what really changes grains from a low-sugar food to a high-sugar food. If you were to take oats in their original form from the field and cook them like rice, you would find that eating oats this way doesn't affect your blood sugar very much. But when you smash those oats and make oatmeal, they increase your blood sugar much more than when you ate them as a whole grain. If you smash the oats even more and make them very thin (now called "quick oats"), then your blood sugar goes up even more.

While you might want to consider having grain such as oatmeal (thick and slow cooked) or brown rice after the six weeks, take the next week (or six weeks) to stay away from all types of grains. The difference in your waistline will be dramatic.

Here is the list of all foods that act like sugars that you should avoid:

- **Grains and grain products**: Rice, corn, wild rice, wheat, barley, oats, and oatmeal, wheat and products made from these grains, including bagels, muffins, cakes, croissants, pancakes, waffles, Pop-Tarts™, donuts, tortillas, English muffins, bread, toast, pasta, cereals, crackers, popcorn, pretzels, any chips (including corn chips, potato chips), grits, polenta, couscous, and many others.
- **Other foods**: French fries or other fried potatoes, pumpkin, Fruit Roll-Ups®, dried dates, all juices, rice milk, jams and jellies, candy or candy bars.

DRAMATIC WEIGHT LOSS

You might find that when you stay away from all sugar and foods that act like sugars that you lose a lot of weight in a short period of time. I've seen this enough to suggest that there may be something else going on other than just losing fat. The most likely scenario is that people are losing fat and water weight.

The reason people lose water is because of a simple body mechanism that can be summed up by the phrase, "The solution to pollution is dilution." What this means is that if you are eating something to which you are allergic, your body holds on to water to protect itself. The body's solution to the pollution (the food to which you are allergic) is to dilute it (hold on to water). I'm not talking about the dramatic bee-sting kind of allergy with these foods, but more of a subtle allergy.

If you find that you lose a lot of weight this week and feel less bloated then you may be one of these people. I mention this here because you should be careful about reintroducing these grains later on. You might find that water weight returns if you decide to eat these grains again. The most likely culprits are wheat and corn: these two grains cause the most allergic reactions and you should be careful if you decide to eat them again. Rice is the safest grain to reintroduce.

NO GRAINS? WHAT CAN I EAT?

While staying away from grains closes down a whole group of foods to you, another opens up. The non-grains such as teff, amaranth, quinoa, and others are great foods to add into your diet. There are some recipes later in the book that include these non-grain foods; you can find others sources of recipes online and in cookbooks. The non-grains are full of nutrition and a great addition to a healthy lifestyle; experiment with them and have fun.

SUGAR ADDICTION

I find the addiction to sugar and foods that act like sugars to be one of the strongest addictions we face. I have a thirty-day program on my website (www.olsonnd.com) that guides people through staying away from sugar and sugary foods for thirty days. The program is a bit more restrictive than I'm suggesting here (for example, you stay away from high glycemic fruits and vegetables such as potatoes). You are welcome to sign up and go through the thirty-day program (there is a free version) while you are going through this program.

Remember to keep up your exercise; this week might be a good week to push yourself a bit and see what you are capable of.

EXPERIMENT NUMBER 4: NO DAIRY

If you are following the plan of adding one new experiment per week, then you should be ready to pick it up a bit by removing all dairy products. Why, you might ask, would you want to remove all dairy products from your diet? The answer is that dairy foods are the highest source of saturated fats in our diets, and, if you are like most people, foods like milk, ice cream, yogurt, butter, and cheese make it to every meal.

You might be thinking that you can switch to skim milk to reduce your fat intake, but skim milk is really no better. As Dr. Joel Fuhrman's points out in his wonderful book, *Eat to Live*, this is a trick of labeling. Milk producers use weight to determine the percentage of fat in their products and this tricks you into thinking you are buying low-fat milk when you actually are not. When you measure the number of calories in whole milk you find out that about half (49 percent) are fat calories. You would expect that skim milk would be less (and it is, but not much). When you measure the number of calories in skim milk, you find out that 35 percent of the calories are fat calories. Take a look:

Milk	Calories	Fat Calories	Percentage
Whole Milk	150	72	49 %
Two Percent	120	45	38 %

There is so-called no-fat milk, but it still has around 4 percent of calories from fat.

WHO DRINKS MILK?

You, of course, have been told your whole life that dairy foods are good for you, but take a look around the world and see if you can find any adult mammal that still consumes milk. You won't find any.

Our addiction to milk and milk products causes us a lot of pain in the long run. Many people are allergic to milk and milk products and are unaware of it. Not only can you be allergic to the sugar in milk (lactose), but you can also be allergic to the proteins in milk. When you are eating something you are allergic to you can produce a large amount of mucus and you tend to gain weight by holding on to water (remember, "the solution to pollution is dilution").

All of this doesn't take into account the large amount of fat that comes with our milk habit. If you want to lose weight, you have to take milk and milk products out of your life. The question "Who drinks milk?" is easily answered: babies. Once you are old enough to read these words, you should stop drinking milk.

WHAT ABOUT CALCIUM?

Whenever I tell someone to stop eating dairy products, the next thing out of his or her mouth is usually, "But where can I get my calcium?" This (as you might have guessed) is just alien advertising. There is an inverse relationship between milk consumption and bone fractures; the more milk products you use the more likely you are to have fractures when you grow old. The countries with the highest consumption of milk are also the countries with the highest percentage of people who have osteoporosis.[51]

While you might think that the only good source of calcium is milk, there are others (many others). Yes, milk does contain calcium (1 cup has 296 mg of calcium), but milk is not the only good source of calcium. Take a look:

- Sesame seeds (1 cup = 702 mg)
- Flax seeds (1 cup = 416 mg)
- Cabbage (1 cup = 380 mg)
- Collard greens (1 cup = 266 mg)
- Spinach (1 cup = 245 mg)
- Oranges (1 cup = 104 mg)
- Kale (1 cup = 94 mg)
- Broccoli (1 cup = 62 mg)

Calcium is abundant in the diet of someone who is eating whole foods. If you are worried about osteoporosis, don't rush out and buy pills with rock calcium in them or drink extra milk; your solution is to eat more leafy green vegetables.

Osteoporosis is a condition that is due to eating a high-fat, high-protein diet along with drinking high phosphorus containing sodas (not your lack of milk). When you are eating a large amount of vegetable matter then you are getting more than enough calcium, plus you are creating an environment where your body is not wasting calcium (this is called acid/base balance). Think about an elephant and how big their bones are; where did they get their calcium? The answer is from the green foods they eat, not from drinking milk. When scientists study bone health, they note that better bones are associated with (you guessed it) eating enough fruits and vegetables, not with the consumption of milk and milk products.[52]

Exercise is also important for preventing osteoporosis, but you are already on a good exercise program so I won't say anything more about that.

MILK SUBSTITUTES

Spend this week not eating any milk or milk products and see how it goes. There are milk substitutes made from soy milk, rice milk, hemp milk, almond milk and coconut milk. My favorite is coconut milk because it contains a fat (a medium-chain fatty acid) that is converted into energy in the body and is not stored as fat. Use these all in small amounts, as all of them (except for rice milk) contain fats. Rice milk should be avoided on this diet; it acts very much like drinking a soda because it is high in simple sugars.

EXPERIMENT NUMBER 5: NO MEAT OR FATS

Just when you thought these crazy experiments couldn't get any harder, I'm going to ask you to take the next step and spend a week without meat or any animal foods; this means you avoid all:

- Chicken, fish, beef, and other animals (this includes eggs)
- Dairy foods including cheese, butter, yogurt, milk

If a food comes from an animal, then don't eat it. You have already removed dairy foods in an earlier step so you are that much closer to successfully completing this step. This experiment removes the largest sources of fats from your diet. The other sources of fat in your diet are those fats found in oils (including any vegetable oils). I am not going to suggest that you take out all vegetable oils from your diet; just use them in moderation. My favorite oils are olive oil and grape seed oil; use as small amounts as you can when cooking. Nuts are another source of good fats; just don't go too crazy with them either (this includes peanut butter). Try to limit yourself to a few handfuls of nuts a day.

There are fats that are essential to your diet (called the essential fatty acids) and you can get these by eating a handful of walnuts a day or by adding flax seeds to your diet.

VEGAN?

Lately there has been a wave of books on becoming vegetarian (no meat diet) or vegan (no meat or dairy products diet) and there is great research that shows that people who eat very little or no meat live longer and healthier lives. I believe that this research to be true and think that you should follow a mostly vegan lifestyle, but I also think that humans are flexible eaters. If you look to our closest relatives (apes) they eat a mostly fruit-based diet, but they also eat meat on occasion. You should follow your ape cousins by eating mostly (90 percent) fruits and vegetables; the remainder of your diet (10 percent) is for eating grains and meats.

I don't want to demonize animal proteins and have you think they are evil. The problem with eating meat is that we eat too much too often. What used to be an occasional meal has become an every-meal event.

This experiment is trying to live without animal proteins for a week or longer. After the program, consider becoming a vegan for most of the week and then occasionally have some meat on your plate on the weekend. What you will find is that a little bit of meat goes a long way when you are not eating it all the time. If you meals are vegetable-focused, then meat becomes a side dish. The best meats to choose are those that are raised as close to their natural environments as possible. This means free-range chickens, beef, and wild fish; game foods such as deer and elk are also a good choice.

SUBSTITUTES

Once again, I'm not big on eating food substitutes, but if you need them for the transition, then use them. There are hamburgers, hot dogs, and all manner of non-meat based foods that look and (kind of) taste like the real thing. Your local health food store will carry these substitutes, but remember that these foods are generally highly processed and full of chemicals so use them moderately.

Beans are another good substitute for people looking for a hearty taste in their meals.

EXPERIMENT NUMBER 6: NO PROCESSED FOODS

If you have been following along and doing a new experiment every week then you are probably very close completing this last experiment, but take the plunge anyway. The experiment for this week is pretty simple: Don't eat anything that comes out of a box, can, or container; or any food that is made in a restaurant.

Most people feel that they don't have time to cook for themselves (and it is true that we all live crazy busy lives) but give it a try anyway. This experiment is designed for you to discover that all you have to do to avoid many of the pitfalls of modern (alien-inspired) eating is to take a little time out of your day and make your own food. As strange as it may sound to you to cook all your own food, your ancestors would be equally puzzled as to why you would let someone else prepare and pre-prepare the foods that you eat.

Prepared food is a modern convenience and one that saves you time, but that ease of food consumption harms both your body and your waistline. The problem with prepared food is that there are too many steps between you and your food. The way I figure it, the more hands and machines that touch your food the worse it is for you.

Think of an apple on a tree. If you go pick that apple and eat it that is the best food you can put in your mouth. If someone else picks that very same apple and it is delivered to you through a grocery store that is not too bad, but still not as good as the self-picked variety. If someone else picks that same apple and then turns it into applesauce then your apple has taken the step into a processed food and has lost vitamins and minerals, depending on how much it has been processed. When food processers get a hold of your apple, they now have the opportunity to add things into your meal that weren't part of the original food (such as sugars, additives, colorings, or preservatives). If your apple was picked and then processed into something like an apple-flavored cereal or apple pie, then you are as far away from that apple you picked on a tree as you can be.

Our bodies pay a heavy price for all of this food processing. We are missing many of the nutrients naturally found in foods when they are processed; nutrients our bodies desperately need. But more importantly, food processers are likely to add sugar, fat, and salt into their foods because that is the only way that they can make us eat them....and we know what happens to sugars and fat in our bodies.

The easiest way to stick to this week's diet is to stay away from any foods that you don't make yourself. Your one exception to the no-processed-foods week is canned foods such as beans, tomatoes, or other vegetables where there is only one ingredient in the can.

I know that you are busy (really, I know) and that you have a million things competing for your time and that we really need to slow down a bit (but that is another book). Making your own food means you are in control of everything that goes into your body. Yes, you can buy foods at a health food store or a healthy restaurant but many of those foods are processed as well. Adding fat, salt, and sugar to foods is something that every company that manufactures food does (no matter what kind of store or restaurant you frequent).

As with everything in this diet, approach this idea of making your own food with an open mind. Give it a try, see what you can do, make gradual improvements all the time.

SIX WEEK OVERVIEW

Here is the whole six week program in review:

- **Week One**: Start exercising and never stop

- **Week Two**: Kick out those added sugars

- **Week Three**: Stay away from the foods that act like sugars

- **Week Four**: Remove dairy from your diet

- **Week Five**: Eliminate meat and other animal product

- **Week Six**: Stop eating all processed foods

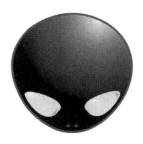

TOOLS FOR THE ROAD LESS
TRAVELED

If you are going to jump on the anti-alien diet, you are definitely headed down the road less traveled. I want you to feel that you can never fail on this diet and that you are just experimenting along the way. You will probably find that the experiments go well some of the times and at other times they do not. If you fall down, just start over again.

Here are some tips to help you navigate through the woods.

WHAT DOES 90 PERCENT
VEGETABLES LOOK LIKE?

Since you are going to drop most animal products and grains out of your life you might be wondering what you are going to replace them with; vegetables are the answer. Remember that your goal is to eat 90 percent of your diet as fruits and veggies. This (admittedly) is a very hard goal to reach but well worth your effort when you start losing weight. While you and your tastes buds might not be happy with your decision to increase the amount of plants that you eat, your body will rejoice at the thought. As your taste buds to adjust to this new diet, vegetables that you thought you would never enjoy will become something you crave (just wait, you will see).

People dislike vegetables for many reasons; sometimes it is as simple as preparing the vegetables correctly. Overcooked green beans are some of the worst food on the planet (at least according to my brother-in-law) but quick roasted green beans with some garlic powder are a great and tasty treat. Learning to cook vegetables correctly is one step to making them a big part of your diet.

Not only are vegetables full of nutrients that your body needs, but they are also low-calorie foods. If you don't currently eat much in the way of the vegetable kingdom, check the list below and see what you can add to your diet. The best vegetables to eat are the leafy green vegetables such as:

Arugula (garden rocket)	Endive	Purslane
Beet greens (spinach beet)	Escarole	Radicchio
	Garden cress	Romaine
Bok Choy	Kale	Sorrel
Borage	Leek	Spinach
Cabbage	Lettuce (all types)	Spring greens
Chard		Turnip greens
Collard greens	Mixed salad greens	Watercress
Dandelion	Mustard greens	

Why are the leafy green veggies the best? The first is that they give your body what it is truly craving: nutrients (vitamins and minerals). The second is that they contain a large amount of fiber, which will make help you to feel full throughout the day. There is an added bonus to having a large amount of leafy green fiber in your diet; fiber helps to move all the junk (especially fat-soluble molecules like cholesterol, hormones, and toxins) out of your body. This fiber sweeping action not only helps your body get rid of stuff it wants to get rid of but it can also help your weight loss.

While it might sound strange right now, include leafy green vegetables with every meal (including breakfast); remember these are all experiments and you will find ways to enjoy the foods that are good for you the more you practice.

Don't forget the rest of the vegetable kingdom and include plenty of the following vegetables:

Acorn Squash	Cucumbers	Pinto beans
Artichoke	Eggplant	Potatoes
Asparagus	Garlic	Pumpkin
Avocado	Green beans	Radish
Azuki beans	Green peppers	Sea vegetables
Beets	Jalapeno peppers	Squash
Black-eyed peas	Leek	Sweet potatoes
Black beans	Lentils	Tomatillo
Broccoli	Lima beans	Tomato
Carrots	Okra	Turnips
Cauliflower	Onion	Yams
Celery	Parsnips	Zucchini
Chickpeas	Peas	

Before we move on, there are three classes of vegetables that deserve special notice. The first is the Brassica vegetables; these include cabbage, broccoli, Brussels sprouts, cauliflower, kale, collards, and mustard greens. These vegetables are remarkable for their ability to prevent diseases such as cancer and other illnesses. They are packed full of nutrients that our bodies crave and need; make sure to add as many of these vegetables to your diet as you can.

Onions and garlic are another super-veggie group; they are a great source of essential nutrients. Both garlic and onions have been studied in a wide variety of diseases (including reducing cholesterol and lowering blood pressure) and they are also great immune-boosting foods. Find a way to sneak onions and garlic into every meal.

Lastly, you should consider the sea vegetables. These vegetables (such as nori, arame, kelp, and others) are full of minerals that we land lubbers are lacking. Experiment with adding the sea vegetables to your diet; they add a nutty, slightly salty taste to most meals.

Variety is the key when it comes to vegetables. Try new vegetables you haven't tried before. The people in the produce section of your store can really help you find new vegetables to try and tips on how to prepare them.

As you might notice, I don't talk much about fruits in this section and that is because experience has taught me that most people who are on this diet will turn to fruits to fill the gap in the loss of sweet things. There are some high sugar fruits such as dates, watermelon, and bananas, but I wouldn't worry too much about those as long as you are not just eating those fruits alone. Once again, try new fruits and vary your diet. Choose the fruits that have the darkest colors (especially the berries: blueberries, blackberries, strawberries), as these are the fruits with the most nutrients that are beneficial for us.

PREPARE TO BE AN ALIEN

I've talked a lot about aliens so far, but what I haven't told you is that YOU are the one who is going to feel like an alien if you follow the advice in this book. All humans are drawn to eat sweet, fatty, and salty food like moths to a flame. We all know how the moth's flame-bound journey ends and our fatty-sweet journey is no different; there is no happy ending to that story.

When you are following this diet and you look around and notice that everyone is eating foods that you are not, you may feel alone. But here is what you need to know: More people are uncovering the alien's evil plan every day and joining you in this battle against unhealthy foods. You won't be alone long. I'm not saying that it will be easy to make the changes you need to make to lose the weight you want to lose and become healthier, but there is a greater payoff that you will find when you look down at your scale, when you discover your energy again, and when you notice how good you look.

If you imagine your life sometime in the future when you have been eating a more plant-based diet and exercising, you will find a different you have arrived at your destination. Change what you are doing right now and you will be placing yourself in a different world, one in which you may never have to deal with heart disease, cancer, or diabetes (much less trying to fit into last year's pants). Think about that. You hold in your hands the opportunity to change the way your life story plays out. Think about not having to be hooked up to an oxygen tank for the last ten years of your life; think about not losing your mind; think about not having to take energy-zapping blood pressure medications; think about not having to inject yourself with insulin, or losing toes and fingers to diabetes. Change your diet today, eat better, lose the weight you want to lose, feel great, and you reduce your chances of ending up a statistic of the ever-growing list of people who are sick, obese, out of shape, and that much closer to an early grave.

Yes, you will feel like an alien if you follow this diet, but the payoff is well worth it.

WHAT TO EXPECT FROM THE RIDE

When you are making changes to your diet, you can expect your body to react. There are two common reactions to making large changes to your diet. The first is that you might feel like you have the flu or a hangover for a while. These are known as withdrawal symptoms (like quitting smoking or drinking alcohol) and for most people the headache and flu-like symptoms are temporary and don't need to be treated.

The second reaction occurs because your body has been waiting patiently for a long time for you to get healthier, so when you start eating better your body views this as a chance to clean house. This healing reaction may cause more prolonged cold-like symptoms or skin conditions like rashes or acne-like eruptions. Don't be alarmed: These symptoms are all temporary and even though it doesn't seem like it, they are signs that you are getting healthier. The best thing you can do is not treat them and let them run their course; make sure you are getting enough rest and drinking enough water. If the symptoms are bad, try this advice:

- **Headaches**: You can use an over-the-counter headache remedy if you like or you can try taking a bit of vitamin C (500 milligrams). Most headaches pass within twenty-four hours of changing your diet. I usually suggest people take Emergen-C, a powder that fizzes when added to water. Yes, Emergen-C does contain some sugar, but I don't expect you to use it for more than a day or two.
- **Diarrhea**: Your body might not be used to digesting all the new and fresh foods you are eating and this can result in diarrhea. Try moving ahead a bit slower and cook most of your food (stay away from raw foods). Your digestion will adapt to a new way of eating soon enough.
- **Constipation**: Constipation is rare on this diet, but does happen. Make sure you are drinking enough water and eating enough fruits and vegetables.
- **Gas and Bloating**: Digestive enzymes can help you deal with the changes in foods you are going through. You might also consider a good probiotic. The gas and bloating symptoms go away when your digestive system adapts to your new way of eating.

Of course, the biggest side effect to this diet is that the weight comes off easily and that you have more energy than that could imagine, so expect that; it is coming.

ALL AT ONCE?

Are you thinking about trying all the experiments at once? That approach can work well for certain people. You know if you are this type of person if you are likely to jump headfirst into a cold pool or the ocean rather than wade in slowly. If you are anxious to get moving on your weight loss then jumping into all the experiments at once is a great idea.

There is some research that supports the idea that it is actually easier to make dramatic changes in your life all at once than to make slow progressive changes over time. You know yourself best so choose the approach that works for you. The rules, though, still apply to you if you are going to go with the all at once approach: All the experiments take practice to be good at; if you fall down then return to the basics.

WHAT ABOUT CAFFEINE?

Both coffee and green tea have more health benefits than not. The only problem with caffeinated substances is that they tend to increase other cravings (like those for sugar). The reason for this is a bit complex but it basically is the result of us trying to self-medicate throughout the day.

If you are typical, you start each day with something sweet and that sugar sends your brain to a happy place (but that happy place doesn't last long). When the effects of breakfast wear off you find yourself needing a boost from coffee. But the opposite is also true: If we get a boost from caffeine and it starts to fade, we reach for sugar to balance our moods. All I can say is you should be careful if you are going to continue drinking coffee and tea and watch how you use them.

I would also suggest that people don't understand how strong their coffee drinks are. I consider coffee to be the hard alcohol of caffeine drinks and that it should only be used in moderation. When people walk into a bar, they don't ask the bartender for a large glass of whisky; they ask for a shot glass. That is because alcohol drinkers know what coffee drinkers don't: that whisky is strong and should only be drunk in small amounts.

When you drink coffee, try drinking it in small cups (like a demitasse) and leave the Tall and Grande sizes for those coffee zombies with the crazed eyes and jittery hands who pass you on the way to the donut house.

WHAT ABOUT CHOLESTEROL?

Cholesterol, it turns out, may be one of the best ways for you to monitor your health. We know cholesterol is a good way to track your overall health because of the largest population study on diet and disease ever conducted. The study, called *The China Study*, followed thousands of people in China and compared their diets to the diseases they were likely to get during their lifetimes. In his book, also called *The China Study*, T. Colin Campbell, PhD confirmed that maintaining a low cholesterol level is closely tied to a reduction in not only heart disease, but also such diverse diseases as diabetes, cancer, and others.

While most doctors suggest that you keep your cholesterol under 200 mg/dL, *The China Study* suggests that your health improves if you keep your cholesterol under 150 mg/dL. But here is the key: You can't get there by taking drugs. Taking cholesterol-lowering drugs has questionable effects on the reduction of heart disease;[53] the only healthy way to lower your cholesterol level is to eat a plant-based diet.

In truth, your cholesterol level should probably fluctuate somewhere between 130 and 180, depending on what you are eating that day. When you have a meal that contains animal protein and fat, your cholesterol will rise; when you have a plant-based meal it will come down.

Consider getting your cholesterol level measured as a way to track how well you are doing on this plan; shoot for a number below 150. As you start to eat a 90 percent fruits and vegetables diet, you will notice your cholesterol levels dropping along with your body weight.

DON'T TRUST YOUR SCALE

The great thing about following a diet is that you can measure your progress along the way. If you are like most people, you have a tool in your house called a scale that will tell you exactly how well you are doing on a diet. The problem with scales is that they lie; they only tell you part of the truth.

The important thing to remember when you step on your scale each morning is that muscle weighs more than fat. If you are following my suggestions for exercise then you are increasing your muscle mass and that can cause some pretty strange things to happen when you take that step on to the scale.

For example: Imagine that before the program you weighed 200 pounds and your body fat was 30 percent. After four weeks following the program perfectly, you again step on the scale. The scale now tells you that you weigh 198 pounds. You might feel like you were wasting your time and that this alien business is nonsense. But if you had a body fat scale (which you can purchase almost anywhere), you would notice that your body fat percentage changed from 30 percent to 26 percent. If that is what happened, then a whole different picture would evolve:

Before Program: You weighed 200 pounds and your body fat was 30 percent

At Four Weeks: You weighed 198 pounds, but your body fat was 26 percent

What has happened? In four weeks, you have lost around nine pounds of body fat! What's more, you have gained six and a half pounds of healthy lean calorie-burning muscle—even though the scale looks almost the same to you. That muscle (as long as you maintain it) will continue to burn and burn and burn calories and that will eventually show up on the scale. Remember that muscles will burn calories as you sleep, when you are awake, and whenever you exercise.

If you really want to track something, track your body fat percentage and not your weight loss; this is especially true for those times when your weight loss slows down.

HOW OFTEN TO EAT

While there is some evidence that eating every few hours helps to keep your blood sugar steady, I'm going to suggest that you try another mini-experiment. For this experiment I want you to wait at least four hours between each of your meals.

The reason for doing this is that so much of what we eat is habit and not hunger. Having something to snack on every few hours is a routine for most people. Eating every four hours is a way to combat your addictions because it is often your addictions driving you to put something in your mouth so often and not true hunger.

Here is the key to eating every four hours: eat as much as you want. As long as you are following a strongly vegetable-based diet, you can eat as much food as you want. What you will find out is that when you eat a lot of vegetables that are full of fiber, you don't crave foods as much as you used to and you feel full. Eating every four hours will help you break those habits that tell you that you need to constantly have something to eat.

RAW FOODS

We are the only animals on this planet who cook their food; that sounds a bit strange, doesn't it? Why do we do that? Cooking foods increases their tastiness and digestibility, but it also decreases their nutritional value (most of the time). There are major differences between eating a raw potato and French fries and the same holds true of other foods that we eat. Raw foods are rich in enzymes, phytonutrients, and antioxidants—all the things you turn to supplements to provide you with and yet they are inside of our foods already (as long as we don't cook them too much). Take a look at all the benefits of eating raw foods:

- Enzymes are the key to good digestion and assimilation of food; raw foods are enzyme rich. Guess what destroys the enzymes in the food we eat? Cooking. It is brilliant that foods contain substances that actually help our bodies break them down and use them. When food is cooked over 118 degrees Fahrenheit, enzymes start to break down and are destroyed. This means that your body has to do all the work.

- Eating raw foods means that you are getting the most out of your food. Vitamins, phytonutrients, and antioxidants are all available to you in raw foods and not left in the oven or on the stovetop.
- Your body tells you when you are full based on two things: the first is if your stomach is full (that is why we should eat so many high-fiber vegetables) and the second is the nutrient value of the food we eat. The more nutrients in the food, the fuller we feel. Have you ever eaten a lot of food but still felt hungry? Chances are the food was overly processed and void of nutrients. You feel fuller faster when you are eating raw, high-nutrient foods.
- There is an immune system reason to eat raw foods. I don't want to freak you out, but raw foods contain bacteria and other microorganisms that stimulate your immune system. This isn't something to be afraid of; it is actually healthy for us. There are theories that suggest that certain conditions, such as asthma, may be the result of living in a too clean environment and that exposure to germs is actually helpful to us.

If you don't eat much in the way of raw foods, work your way slowly into it (over months). You want to eat as many raw foods as you can, but start with adding a salad or mixed greens to most of your meals or try snacking on raw carrots, apples, berries, and other fruits.

MOTIVATION

Motivation is a strange animal that tends to visit you at odd times during your life. Ask what you should do to stay motivated and you might as well ask how to stay motivated to stay motivated.

I find that the best way to stay motivated is to surround yourself with other people who have the same goals in mind that you do. You can help yourself by reading books similar to this one (check the resources section at the end of the book), or by connecting with people who are also looking to lose weight and become healthier. You can also find people in your life who are in the same place and going down the same road as you are. But don't stop there; you can try making a competition out of following this diet while someone else joins you or even follows another diet. For some people it helps to put money on the line (even small amounts) that you pay if you don't meet your goals.

The online world also offers many places to connect. You can stop by the website for this book (www.thealiendiet.com) anytime you want to connect with other people and get help with your own journey. You can join the group on Facebook that focuses on this book or my 30 Sugar Free Days Program (see the resource section).

One of the best ways to stay motivated is to measure your progress but remember to not fall into the trap of using a scale as your only means of measuring your progress (think body fat percentage and cholesterol levels). Weight is certainly one measuring tool but it can lie to you as you gain much-needed muscle mass when you start exercising. One of the best tools to measure your progress is a body composition scale. These scales measure your body fat and lean protein mass. You want to see your body fat drop and an increase in your lean protein mass as you progress through the weeks.

Another great motivational tool is to choose a race or some athletic event. Some people go crazy and decide to run marathons but a shorter race can be a great goal as well (you can choose to walk most 5K and 10K races—check for one in your local area). Having a race like that in front of you helps get you out of bed in the morning and on the trail.

Motivation comes and goes and that is very natural. The more tools you have at your side, the better and easier it will be for you.

CHEATING

What is the best way to go through the whole program? Don't cheat at all.

Having said that, most people have a hard time envisioning eating this way for the rest of their lives. For them, I suggest that you try (like you did in high school) to get an "A" in nutrition. You are an A student by becoming a 90-percent-non-grain-super-vegetable-eating-vegan-athlete. If you continue this diet in a 90 percent way you will still be getting the benefits of it and allowing yourself to stray now and them.

The question then becomes: What does that look like? There is really no answer for everyone, but say you really want a large chunk of meat then go ahead and have it. If that birthday cake tempts you then cut yourself a slice.

What you are going to find if you stray is one of two things. The first is that you didn't enjoy that food as much as you thought you would. That cake or steak isn't going to taste as good as you remembered. You may learn that it is not worth it to stray and that temporary sensation of pleasing your mouth pales in comparison to how bad you feel. This is especially true for people when they try eating processed foods again: they find that they feel terrible or that they wake up the next morning sluggish and in a bad mood. Look on these moments as "learning from your body moments" and understand that your body is helping you to a better way to live.

The other possibility is that you stray from the diet and then start binging on all the food you used to eat. This can potentially lead to you regaining the all the weight you lost. Remember that this is a part of the process too. If you fall down, pick yourself up again. Use your resources at the end of the book; find another book, some more friends, or a group that will help keep you motivated.

When you decide to cheat, I suggest that you choose one thing at a time and see how you do. You may find that oatmeal in the morning is fine for you, but that drinking a soda makes you feel like a slug. Ultimately your body will tell you what works for you and what doesn't; take the time to listen.

HOW LONG SHOULD YOU STAY ON THE DIET?

Six weeks is a good stretch of time to test out the diet and think about reintroducing some of the foods you have been missing. My hope is that you embrace this kind of diet for the rest of your life and see it as a process and not a destination. Maybe last week you were getting an "A" in nutrition, but this week you are getting a "C". If this happens, just view the next week as your chance to start over again. Remember, if you are focusing on your health then your weight naturally normalizes.

One of the hardest things to accept about a change in lifestyle is that your journey is not a straight one. You are likely to lose a ton of weight the first few weeks on this diet but that amount of weight loss isn't likely to continue in a straight line. You might lose the most weight in the first few weeks and then not lose a bunch until the twelfth or thirteenth week (our bodies are strange that way).

You also may find it easy to stay on the diet for weeks or months but then slip and start eating junk again. This is actually more normal than people staying on a diet like this for the rest of their lives (most people slide back at least a little bit).

Settle in for a lifetime; keep coming back to the experiments and see if you learn something new the next time around. This isn't a diet you are on until you lose weight; this diet is what your body needs to function at its best and should be a lifetime pursuit. You learn how to do it better the longer that you try. Take your slip-ups as part of the journey; as you learn more about what to cook, how to eat, and what to avoid, your slip-ups become fewer and fewer. When you arrive at the weight you want to be at then that occasional piece of chocolate cake will make no difference (remember, you are just trying to get an "A," not be perfect).

Most people have a hard time avoiding grains for the rest of their lives; try whole foods versions of grains such as brown rice and slow-cooked oatmeal (not quick oats). The occasional tortilla or bread won't hurt you too much either as long as your diet is predominately vegetable-based.

WHERE ARE YOU HEADED?

It is a good idea to know where you are going when you start on a journey. While some of the experiments are meat-free weeks or grain-free weeks this doesn't mean that you have to abandon these foods forever. It means that they should be regulated to the place in our diets where they belong: small amounts are okay; large amounts are not.

Most people eat diets that are 80 percent meat and grain and 20 percent fruits and vegetables; this is the opposite of the way you should be eating. A diet that is 20 percent meat and grains and 80 percent fruits and vegetables is what you are looking for; or if you are really committed, kick that up to 90 percent fruits and vegetables.

You want to get as close as you can to eating the optimal diet for humans, which means eating mostly fruits, vegetables, and beans and eating a small amount of grains and meats. Once you make the transition to a plant-based diet, it is best to leave dairy products out of your life for good, but this is an individual choice.

Each step you make toward eating more vegetables, the better you will feel and the more weight you will lose. You might find that you quickly adapt to this way of eating and that you enjoy the energy and weight loss that come from eating the way humans are supposed to eat. You may also find that you adapt to certain parts of the diet easily, while others are harder (maybe kicking dairy was no problem, but staying away from grains is difficult—or vice versa). That is what the experiments are for; simply pick a week and go back to the experiment with which you are having problems and see if you learn anything new about how you can avoid the food in the experiment.

Ultimately you will have good weeks and bad weeks; both are okay as long as the long-term push is toward better eating. I've said this enough throughout the book, but it is really important: If you feel like you are slipping then simply try an experiment (or all of them) for seven days, twenty-one days, or thirty days.

Good luck on your journey to a healthier you!

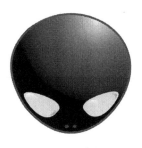

WHAT TO EAT

The following recipes are all grain-free, dairy-free, sugar-free and meat-free and meet the requirements of all the experiments. Feel free to make adjustments to the recipes, depending on what stage you are at.

In the following recipes I mention the use of coconut milk often. This is the coconut milk that comes in a carton similar to cow's milk and is made by a company called So Delicious (you can find this in most health foods stores) and you should choose the no-sugar kind. If the recipe requires the more traditional type of coconut milk (much thicker) then it says use a *can* of coconut milk.

BREAKFAST

Breakfast is probably the hardest meal for most people because we have been trained that we have to eat something sweet in the morning. And that is exactly why it is the most important meal of the day. If you start out your morning eating something sweet, then you are going to want to eat something sugary throughout the rest of the day (I call this the sugar-magnet effect: once you put some sugar in your body, more wants to follow it).

In my house we tend to lean on dinner leftovers for breakfast, we also do smoothies, chili and even simply just fruit.

BEANS

Beans for breakfast? The answer is yes! Beans not only help you to feel full throughout the day, they actually help to balance your blood sugar. How should you prepare them? Try Dr. Scott's chili recipe later on in this section, but also try whole or refried beans. For an occasional cheat (once you are through the six weeks), try using rice or wheat tortillas along with refried beans, salsa and lettuce or baby greens mix. You can also try brown rice, beans and vegetables.

SMOOTHIES

Smoothies and shakes are a great way to start the day. They give you the sweet taste you are probably used to and they are packed full of great nutrients (especially if you are using a lot of berries).

The liquid portions of these smoothies often call for a milk substitute. My favorite milk substitute is coconut milk (this is not the small cans of coconut milk that you may be familiar with, but is found in the refrigerator section of a health food store); the brand I like is called SO Delicious. You can also use rice milk or almond milk. Rice milk is very sweet, so use it in moderation and I'm not a big fan of soy milk, but you can use it if you like it.

Make sure you choose the unsweetened versions of these milk substitutes.

All of these smoothies push the envelope of being too sugar-like, but the sugars can be balanced by the protein, fibers in the fruits and the fat found in almond, soy or coconut milk. Focus on using low-sugar fruits such as the berries (strawberries, blueberries, blackberries, raspberries) and keep the bananas to a minimum.

BASIC SMOOTHIE RECIPE

Make it the way you like it.

1/4 cup juice (apple, cranberry...)
1/4 banana
1/2 cup frozen berries (strawberries, raspberries, blueberries)
1/2 cup unsweetened coconut milk (or rice or almond milk)
1 scoop protein powder (hemp, rice, pea or soy)

Add in any other fresh or frozen fruit you like: peaches, apples, grapes... Combine all the ingredients in a blender or food processor and blend until smooth. You may have to add more juice or coconut milk depending on your frozen ingredients and your blender.

FROZEN AVOCADO SHAKE

This shake sounds a bit strange, but give it a try.

1/4 cup juice (apple, cranberry...)
1/4 cup mashed avocado
1/4 banana, mashed
1/2 cup fresh or frozen strawberries
1/2 cup unsweetened coconut milk (or rice or almond milk)
1/2 tsp. almond or vanilla extract

Combine all the ingredients in a blender or food processor and blend until smooth. You may have to add more juice or coconut milk depending on your frozen ingredients and your blender.

DATE SHAKE

Dates are naturally high in sugar, so use this drink as an occasional treat.

1 cup rice, almond or coconut milk
12 pitted dates, chopped
6 almonds
1 cup plain coconut or soy yogurt
1/2 cup unsweetened coconut milk (or rice or almond milk)
4 ice cubes

Combine all the ingredients in a blender or food processor and blend until smooth. You may have to add more juice or coconut milk depending on your frozen ingredients and your blender.

SAUCES AND DIPS

Sauces can be a wonderful addition to any meal, but are hard to make without wheat, rice, or dairy. Check out the following sauces that meet the requirements of all the experiments.

CURRY SAUCE

2 Cups water or coconut milk
1/4 - 1/2 cups potato flour
1/4 cup nutritional yeast
1-2 tablespoons miso
1 teaspoon garlic powder
1-2 teaspoons curry powder

Combine all ingredients into a blender or food processer. Pour the mixture into a saucepan and gently heat. The potato flour is the thickener and you can add more, but only when you mix it with a bit of water first (it will often clump if you add it to the hot mixture – if this happens, return it to the blender and then back to the saucepan).

PEA GUACAMOLE

Yes, you can make guacamole from peas and it is mighty tasty!

2 cups frozen sweet peas, thawed
1 tomato, chopped
1/4 cup finely chopped red onions
1/4 cup chopped fresh cilantro
2 tablespoons green chili peppers (chopped)
2 tablespoons lime juice
1/2 teaspoon ground cumin
Olive oil
Salt and pepper to taste

Place peas, lime juice, onions and cilantro into a food processer and process until smooth. Transfer to a bowl and mix in the remaining ingredients. The color will fade if you leave this out, so eat it soon after making.

MUSHROOM GRAVY

Here is a gravy that tastes good on a lot of vegetables besides potatoes. I like portabella mushrooms, but you can use shitake or even standard "medium" mushrooms you find in your local store.

1-2 cups mushrooms
1 medium onion
2-3 cloves garlic
1/8 – 1/4 cup potato flour
1 tablespoon miso
1/8 cup nutritional yeast

1/2 cup vegetable broth
Olive oil
Soy sauce to taste

Dice onions and garlic into small pieces. Sauté the onions in a little olive oil until tender, allowing the onion to brown a little. Add in garlic and let sauté for a few minutes. Add in the rest of the ingredients and whisk until smooth. The key here is to get a thick gravy and this may take adding in more potato flour or more vegetable broth to get the consistency that you want.

HUMMUS AND VEGGIES

Hummus is one of the few mixed foods that have been tested and shown to be low on the glycemic index. You can now buy hummus at most grocery stores, but here is a recipe you can try:

16 oz can of chickpeas
3-5 tablespoons lemon juice
2 tablespoons tahini (sesame butter)
2 cloves garlic, crushed
1/2 teaspoon salt
2 tablespoons olive oil

Place all contents into blender or food processer; use the juice from the garbanzo beans to make smooth. Enjoy the hummus as a dip for any fresh vegetables (broccoli, carrots, cauliflower, celery) you like.

MANGO SALSA

Ready for a high nutrient and great tasting salsa? Try this mango salsa.

1 ripe mango, peeled and diced
1 tablespoon finely chopped jalapeno

1 small diced onion (red or white)
1 tablespoon lime juice
Cilantro leaves to taste
Salt and pepper to taste

Mix ingredients together in a bowel for chunky salsa or lightly blend ingredients for a smoother salsa.

SALADS

I'm guessing that you know how to make a salad, but here are a few combinations you may not have thought about.

SESAME AND GARLIC SPINACH

Here is a great cooked salad. You can also try it with other greens such as kale, arugula or escarole.

4-6 cloves garlic
6-8 cups baby spinach
1/8 teaspoon red pepper flakes
1/2 cup water
Sesame seeds
Olive oil
Salt to taste

Sauté the garlic in olive oil until tender. Add in red pepper flakes and spinach, plus water. Let the water steam the spinach until wilted. Serve with a topping of sesame seeds.

BEAN SALAD

This is a great summer salad. Choose fresh vegetables from your garden or local farmer's market.

1 small red onion
1/8 cup apple cider vinegar
1 15-ounce can pinto or white beans
2 tablespoons fresh parsley
2 tablespoons fresh chives
1/4 cup olive oil
Salt to taste

Dice the onions and drain the water off of the beans and mix all the ingredients together. To this basic mixture add in whatever is fresh. Try Green beans, broccoli, peas or other garden vegetable. You can put the vegetables in the salad raw or lightly steam them before mixing.

GRILLED VEGETABLE SALAD

Once again, choose any vegetables that you like.

1 small eggplant
1 zucchini
1 red bell pepper
1 small onion
2 teaspoons red wine vinegar
1/4 teaspoon basil
Olive oil
Salt and pepper

Slice the eggplant into thick rounds and soak in a bowl of salt water for 20 minutes. Cut the rest of the vegetables into thick rounds. Drain eggplant and mix in a bowl with olive oil and pepper. Grill the vegetable on a grill pan. Drizzle with vinegar and sprinkle basil over the top.

QUINOA SALAD

Quinoa is one of the few grains allowed on this diet. It is actually not a grain at all, but classified as a seed and what a seed it is! Packed full of nutrients, quinoa adds a nutty flavor to any dish. Make sure you wash it before you use it as this removes the bitter taste that sometimes is associated with quinoa.

4 cups vegetable broth
2 cups quinoa
1 cucumber
1 red bell pepper
2 garlic cloves
1 cup broccoli
2 tomatoes
2-3 tablespoons lemon juice
Olive oil
Salt and pepper to taste

Place vegetable broth and quinoa in a saucepan and bring to a boil. Cover and reduce the temperature to simmer. Cook until done (usually around 20 minutes). Slice cucumber, bell pepper, garlic, broccoli and tomatoes. Add vegetables and olive oil into pot and stir. Allow to cool and season with salt and pepper.

SHALADA BRANIYA

This is a Moroccan eggplant cooked salad.

1 large eggplant
4-6 cloves garlic, minced
1 large tomato
4-6 cups water or vegetable broth
2 teaspoons cumin
1 teaspoon paprika
1/8 teaspoon cayenne
4 tablespoons lemon juice

ARE ALIENS MAKING **YOU FAT?**

2 tablespoons olive oil
Chopped fresh coriander
Salt and pepper to taste

Cut the eggplant into cubes and place it in a large saucepan along with the minced garlic and 1 teaspoon of salt. Let gently boil covered for 5-10 minutes, or until eggplant is cooked, but still firm. Drain using a strainer (you don't want to lose the garlic) and place into a salad bowl. Mix the remaining spices, lemon juice and olive oil into the bowl. Serve with a topping of fresh coriander.

SOUPS AND CHILIES

The benefits of soup are endless: low cooking temperatures preserve nutrients; any nutrients leaving the vegetables end up in the broth and the high amounts of vegetables and water are exactly what your body is craving.

Soups fill you up more than you think. In a recent study, participants were divided into two groups. The first was put on a limited diet. The second group was put on the same diet, but told to eat two bowls of soup a day. At the end of a year, the two groups lost about the same amount of weight, what was the difference? The group that ate two bowels of soup felt much more full and satisfied. How would you like to spend a year? Hungry or satisfied?

In our house, we tend to make chili a lot and store it for the next week so that it is available when we are hungry and need something quick.

DR. SCOTT'S CHILI

Around our house, this is an every-morning meal (yes, we eat this for breakfast). We usually make a large batch of chili and stick it in the refrigerator so that we have it whenever we need it.

1 (30 ounce can) tomato puree
1 (6 ounce can) tomato paste
1 (4 ounce can) diced jalapeno peppers
1 (4 ounce can) diced green chili peppers
1 (30 ounce can) Pinto or Black beans
1 (large) onion
2-3 potatoes, grated
3 stalks of celery, grated
1 sweet potato, grated
2-3 cloves garlic
2 Tablespoons cumin
1 Tablespoon coriander
1/2 Tablespoon paprika
2 Tablespoons parsley

Set entire ingredients in Crockpot and cook on medium to high for 4 to 6 hours.

SWEET POTATO AND TOMATO SOUP

We add in the skins of the sweet potatoes, but you can peel them before adding them in to the dish.

2 or 3 large sweet potatoes, diced
1 15 ounce can of tomato sauce
1 or 2 red onions
2 or 3 cloves of garlic
Olive oil
Salt and pepper to taste

Cover the garlic and onions with olive oil and gently simmer until tender. Add the tomato sauce and chopped sweet potatoes. Simmer until potatoes are tender, add water if necessary. Blend in a blender or food processer, return to the pot and cook for 10 or so minutes. For an interesting taste, try roasting the garlic in the oven before adding it to the soup.

BUTTERNUT SOUP

This basic soup is great. For an extra tasty version, try replacing one cup of the water with one can of coconut milk.

1 butternut squash
4-6 cups water
1 onion, chopped
4 cloves of garlic, chopped
Olive oil
Salt and pepper

Cut and deseed the squash. Cover the onion and garlic with olive oil and gently simmer until tender. Add the squash and onions to a large pot and cover with water. Bring to a boil and then reduce to a simmer. Flavor with your favorite spices, we like cumin, coriander, oregano, basil and sometimes cayenne pepper. Blend in a blender or food processer, return to the pot and cook for 10 or so minutes.

CARROT COCONUT SOUP

Carrots and coconut are the perfect combination any time of year.

4-6 large carrots
1 large yellow onion
Olive oil
Salt to taste
1 teaspoon fresh ginger
2 teaspoons curry powder
14 ounce can of coconut milk
1-2 cups water or vegetable broth

Cover the onions with olive oil and gently simmer until tender. Add in the rest of the ingredients (except for the coconut milk) and simmer for 30 minutes. Add in coconut milk and blend in a blender or food processer, return to the pot and cook for 10 or so minutes.

BLACK BEAN SOUP

Black bean soup is one of my all time favorites, especially during cold winter months. We use a whole bulb of garlic in this recipe, but use as much as you like.

2 15-ounce cans black beans
1 16-ounce can vegetable broth
2-4 cloves of garlic
1 large red or yellow onion
1-2 stalks celery
Olive oil
2 teaspoons cumin
1 tablespoon chili powder
Black pepper and salt

Cover the onion and garlic with olive oil and gently simmer until tender. Pour both cans of beans into medium saucepan. Add vegetable broth, celery, and seasonings. Bring to a boil and let simmer until celery softens. Take out 1/2 of the soup and puree in a blender or food processor and then return to the pot, let cook for another 10 minutes or so. Garnish with fresh cut onion and cilantro or corn.

LENTIL CHILI WITH CUMIN AND GREEN ONIONS

Unlike other beans, lentils cook up quickly. There are all sorts of varieties of lentils, try the green, brown or even red lentils for this recipe.

1 cup dried lentils
4 cups water or vegetable broth
1 30-ounce can tomato puree (or sauce)

2 tsp olive oil
1 medium onion
3 garlic cloves
2 Tbsp chili powder
1 Tbsp ground cumin
1 tsp dried oregano leaves
1/8 tsp cayenne pepper

Add water and lentils to a large pot and bring to a light boil for 20-30 minutes. Add the rest of the ingredients and reduce to a simmer for another 30 minutes. If you like thick chili, let the water boil off, if you like thinner, then add more. You can thicken up the chili by blending 1/2 of the chili in a blender or food processer. Try adding chopped fresh green onions to the pot right before serving.

POTATO BROCCOLI SOUP

Deliciously satisfying, this soup is easy to make and gets better the longer you have it. It contains nutritional yeast, which you can find at your local health food store.

Six medium Yukon gold potatoes
1 bunch broccoli
1-2 stalks of celery
1 Large yellow onion
4-6 cloves garlic
1/4 cup nutritional yeast
Salt to taste

Chop and combine all ingredients in a large pot or crockpot. Bring to a boil and let simmer slowly until potatoes are cooked. Blend in a food processor or blender until smooth. Try keeping out 1/2 of the broccoli and then adding it to the soup after blending.

LENTIL SWEET POTATO SOUP

This one takes a bit more time, but is well worth the effort.

1 cup brown lentils
4-6 cups water or vegetable broth
2-3 medium sweet potatoes or yams
1-2 celery stalks
2-4 garlic cloves
1 green pepper (or 1/2 green, 1/2 red)
1-2 jalapeno peppers
1 6-ounce can of tomato paste
1 tablespoon cumin
1/2 teaspoon dried thyme
1 teaspoon basil
1 teaspoon paprika
1 teaspoon coriander
1/2 teaspoon fennel
Olive oil
Salt & pepper to taste

Add the lentils to a large soup pot along with water or vegetable broth; bring to a boil then let cook at a low boil for 30 minutes. Sauté celery, garlic, green and jalapeno peppers in olive oil until soft. Chop sweet potatoes and add them to the pot along with the rest of the ingredients. Cook at a low temperature for another 30 minutes.

MOROCCAN VEGGIE STEW

1 butternut squash
2 medium carrots
1 large onion
1 cup chopped celery
1 15-ounce can garbanzo beans
1 15-ounce can diced tomatoes
1/2 cup raisins

1 tablespoon ground cumin
1 tablespoon dried parsley
1/2 teaspoon ground cinnamon
1/8 to 1/4 teaspoon red pepper flakes
Vegetable broth
Olive oil
Salt and pepper to taste

Saute onion in olive oil until soft. Combine all ingredients in large pot and add enough vegetable broth and water to cover the vegetables. Bring to a boil and lower to a simmer for 40 minutes.

LENTIL MUSHROOM SOUP

Mushrooms (like Shitake, Maitake and others) are packed full of great nutrients, and they taste good.

2-3 large Portobello mushrooms
4-6 Shitake mushrooms
2 cups lentils
1 green bell pepper
1 large onion
4 cloves garlic
1 (6 ounce) can tomato paste
4-6 cups water or vegetable broth
Olive oil
1 teaspoon dried basil and/or oregano
Salt and pepper to taste

Add four cups of water to a large pot and cook the lentils for 1/2 hour. Chop onions, garlic, bell pepper and mushrooms and sauté them with enough olive oil to keep them from sticking. Combine all ingredients in the soup pot and simmer for 1/2 hour (add extra water if needed). Blend 1/2 of ingredients in a food processor or blender to thicken and then return to the pot.

POTATO, LENTIL AND CAULIFLOWER SOUP

This soup is really smooth and creamy.

2 large potatoes
1 large head of cauliflower
2 stalks celery
1 cup lentils
1 large onion
4 to 6 cloves garlic
2 cups chopped spinach or kale
4-6 cups water
Olive oil
1/2 can of coconut milk
2 tablespoons curry powder
1/2 teaspoon ground turmeric
1/2 teaspoon oregano
1/4 teaspoon lemon juice
Salt and pepper to taste

Add four cups of water to a large pot and cook the lentils for 1/2 hour. Chop celery, potatoes, onions and garlic and add to the pot. Add spices and coconut milk to the pot; simmer on medium heat for another 1/2 hour. Blend all of the ingredients in a food processor or blender to thicken and then return to the pot. Gently stir in spinach or kale and cook for another 10 minutes.

SWEET POTATO, APPLESAUCE AND CURRY SOUP

Applesauce is not the first thing you think about putting in a soup, but it gives this wonderful soup a creamy texture.

2-3 sweet potatoes
1 medium onion
2-4 cloves of garlic
1 cup of no-sugar applesauce

4-6 cups water or coconut milk
1/2 teaspoon dried ginger
1/4 teaspoon nutmeg
2 teaspoons curry powder
Olive oil

Sauté onions and garlic until soft. Combine in a large pot the sweet potatoes and the rest of the ingredients. Cover with water or coconut milk. Bring to a boil and simmer until potatoes are soft and then blend in a food processer or blender to thicken and return to the pot. Simmer for another 20 minutes and serve.

ANY TIME

ROASTED VEGGIES

While veggies are best when they are raw, every once in a while you need something more hearty

Choose any of the following veggies you enjoy and chop them into small pieces:

Asparagus
Broccoli
Brussels sprouts
Cabbage
Carrots
Cauliflower
Green beans
Green Peas
Garlic
Onion
Potatoes
Sweet potato

Place the veggies into a Pyrex cooking pan and pour the following mixture over the top:

1-2 tablespoons dry curry or other spice you like
1 teaspoon salt
2- Tablespoons olive oil

Bake at 350 degrees Fahrenheit for 25-35 minutes.

TEMPEH WITH COCONUT MILK

Tempeh is another soy based food, it is like tofu but more chewy and (some say) meat-like.

1 pound tempeh
1 red bell pepper
1 cup snow peas
1 onion
1 can coconut milk
1/4 cup no-sugar peanut butter
4 Tablespoons soy sauce
2 Tablespoons minced lemongrass
1 teaspoon crushed red pepper (optional)
Olive oil
Juice of 1 lime
1/4 cup peanuts

Cut onions, bell peppers, snow peas and tempeh and stir fry for 3-5 minutes. Combine coconut milk, peanut butter, soy sauce and crushed red pepper into a blender and blend until smooth. Add sauce to vegetable mixture and simmer for five minutes. Mix in lime juice and garnish with peanuts.

LENTIL LOAF

Lentil loaf is a standard staple among the meatless crowd and a hearty meal for anyone.

1 cup brown lentils
1-2 cloves garlic
1 small carrot
1 stalk celery
1 small red bell pepper
1 small can tomato paste
Olive oil
1-2 tablespoons soy sauce
1/8 cup nutritional yeast
1 Tablespoon fresh ginger
1 teaspoon coriander
1 teaspoon paprika
1/2 teaspoon rosemary
1/2 teaspoon thyme
Salt and pepper to taste

Cover lentils in water and bring to a boil, simmer at medium to low heat for an hour until thoroughly cooked. Drain lentils and place in a bowl. Chop vegetables and grate carrots. Sauté garlic for five minutes and then add in the rest of the vegetables. Place contents in a small loaf pan and cook at 350 degrees For 45 minutes.

Try adding in chopped broccoli or grated potato, sweet potato, or your favorite vegetables.

GRILLED MANGOS

Never had grilled mangos? Then you are in for a treat.

3-4 mangos
1 lime
Olive oil

Salt, pepper and cayenne to taste
Jalapeno peppers
Cilantro

Peel and cut the mangos into large flat slices and place on a cookie sheet or other flat surface. Sprinkle with olive oil, salt, pepper and cayenne. Grill the seasoned mango slices for 1-2 minutes on each side. Squeeze fresh lime juice on top and garnish with chopped cilantro and jalapeno peppers.

You can top this with a cream-like substitute (though this can be high fat)

1 cup coconut or other milk substitute
1/4 cup grapeseed oil
1 teaspoon vanilla extract
1-2 teaspoons guar gum

SWISS CHARD AND GARBANZOS

2 Large bunches of Swiss chard
2 15-ounce cans garbanzo beans
1 cup chopped red onions
1-2 cloves garlic
2 tablespoons tomato paste
1 teaspoon ground cumin
1/2 cup chopped fresh parsley
Olive oil
Salt to taste

Take the stems out of the Swiss chard and chop the leaves. Place the leaves in boiling salt water for about 5 minutes. Drain water. Sauté onions and garlic. Mix in a bowl the rest of the ingredients and stir in the cooked chard.

KALE, QUINOA, AND MUSHROOMS

1 cup quinoa
2 small sweet potatoes
1 cup mushrooms (shitake, Maitake…)
2 cloves garlic
1 bunch kale
1 cup vegetable broth
Olive oil
kosher salt and black pepper
Nutritional yeast

Cook quinoa by first washing quinoa and then adding two cups of water and the quinoa to a saucepan and bring to a boil, let simmer for 20 minutes. Chop and sauté the garlic in another saucepan. Chop the mushrooms and add to the garlic mixture. Cut the sweet potatoes into small chunks so that they cook quickly and add them to the mixture. Sauté for 10 to 15 minutes and then add in vegetable broth and cooked quinoa. Cut the kale into small pieces and mix into dish.

Place all ingredients in a blender and blend. The thickener is the guar gum and it takes a while to thicken, so blend and then wait and see if it is thick enough. Add more guar gum if you need it. Having a hard time finding guar gum? Try other thickeners such as xanthan gum or even tapioca flour.

NO GRAIN NOODLES AND SAUCE

How do you make noodles without grains? Raw food enthusiasts are using carrots (see Ani Phyo's Ani's Raw Food Essentials) and jicama (see Lisa Mann's The World Goes Raw Cookbook), but I think the best are made from squash. Try any of the below combinations.

NOODLES:

Spaghetti squash: cut one medium to large spaghetti squash lengthwise and scoop out seeds. Bake in oven at 350 until soft (usually around 30 minutes). When you scoop out the meat of the squash, it looks like spaghetti.

Zucchini: peel off the outer skin of the zucchini and then using a vegetable peeler; cut wide ribbons of zucchini (too look like fettuccine). You may have to slice them lengthwise if you like a smaller noodle. Place your noodles into a colander and sprinkle with salt. Let drain for 30 minutes.

SAUCE:

Choose any sauce you like such as tomato sauce or pesto. We like garlic (lightly simmered in olive oil) and broccoli. Choose whatever you have around the house: nuts, tomatoes, avocado, asparagus…

EGGPLANT AND TOFU

I'm not a big fan of tofu and tempeh (meat substitutes), but they are great for the occasional meal, and this meal is delicious.

1 pound of firm tofu
2 large eggplants
6-8 cloves of garlic
2 tablespoons tomato paste
Soy sauce to taste (about 3 tablespoons)
1 teaspoon hot chili sauce
2 tablespoons grated ginger
3 tablespoons rice vinegar
Sesame oil

Cut the eggplant into long strips and marinate it in a bowel with the tomato paste, chili sauce, ginger and rice vinegar for 10-15 minutes and then place the eggplant in a skillet or wok with a little soy sauce and sesame oil, and cook gently until eggplant is soft. Drain the water out of the tofu and let it rest on a cutting board for 10-15 minutes (this takes a lot of the water out). Cut tofu into small, long strips. In a skillet, heat the tofu along with about 3 tablespoons of sesame oil and 3 tablespoons of soy sauce. Brown the tofu on both sides, then add the tofu to the eggplant mixture and gently stir (tofu falls apart easily).

FAJITAS

I know what you are thinking: there is no way vegetable based fajitas taste anywhere as good as the meat kind, but give these a try, they are great. While any vegetables will do for this recipe, I've included some that I think work best.

Marinade:
1/4 cup olive oil
1/4 cup red wine vinegar
1 teaspoon oregano
1 teaspoon chili powder
1-3 teaspoons garlic powder
Salt and pepper to taste

Vegetables (choose what you like):
Zucchini
Yellow squash
Onion
Bell peppers (try red, green and yellow)
Mushrooms (try portabella, shitake)
Broccoli
Cauliflower
Carrots

Mix together marinade and set aside. Cut vegetables into thin strips and let soak in marinade for at least 1/2 hour or overnight. Cook in a hot pan with a little bit of olive oil or grapeseed oil. Serve with beans, avocado. If you are a fan of eggplant, try that too!

BEAN BURGERS

If you are missing a good burger, these won't quite take the place, but pretty close. You can use all the same beans or mix them (pinto, black, kidney, garbanzo...)

6 cans of beans
1 small onion
2 carrots
1 medium potato
1 teaspoon garlic powder
1 teaspoon onion powder
1 teaspoon chili powder
2 teaspoons ground cumin

Drain the beans and mash with a potato masher in a large bowl. Dice the onions and grate the carrots and potato and combine with the beans. Mix in spices and then form into balls. Flatten the balls onto a cookie sheet and bake at 350 for 20 minutes or until done.

GARBANZO BURGERS

Quick and easy substitutes for traditional burgers.

16 oz can garbanzo or chickpeas, drained
1/2 cup onions, chopped
1-2 cloves of garlic
1 tsp ground cumin

1 tsp fresh ground black pepper
1/4 tsp sea salt
2 tbsp soy sauce

Mash the ingredients by hand, or use a food processor. Form the mixture into individual patties and then place on a non-stick pan and cook at 350 degrees for 20 minutes or until done. If you are really missing crispy food, these can also be fried on a stovetop.

Need a non-grain bun? Try using lettuce leaves. We enjoy these burgers plain with salsa and mashed avocado on top.

VEGGIE KABOBS

The possibilities are endless!

Choose any fruit or vegetable you like (that will hold up on a grill)

Tomatoes
Mushrooms
Zucchini
Bell peppers
Summer squash
Asparagus
Onions
Tofu
Pineapple
Mango
Peaches

Place all the veggies in a bowel and then try these marinades:

Simple: Salt, pepper, olive oil
Simple Plus: Salt, pepper, olive oil, garlic powder, onion powder also try cayenne, cumin

Teriyaki:
1/4 cup soy sauce
1/4 cup rice wine or sake
2 tablespoons rice vinegar
2 tablespoons honey
2 cloves garlic chopped fine
1-2 teaspoons minced ginger root
Sesame oil

(Yes, this Teriyaki sauce has honey in it. I have tried to make a non-sugar teriyaki sauce, but it just didn't work. The amount of sugar in this sauce is so small that the apple you ate this morning has more sugar in it)

Herb:
1/2 cup olive oil
1/4 vinegar or lemon juice
2 garlic cloves, minced
1 teaspoon Dijon mustard
1/2 teaspoon dried basil
1/2 teaspoon dried oregano
1/2 teaspoon dried rosemary
Salt and pepper to taste

STUFFED PEPPERS

Try using all different colored bell peppers (green, red, yellow) to make this dish even more colorful.

4 bell peppers
1 yellow onion
1 red onion
2-4 cloves of garlic
2 stalks celery
2 medium carrots
1/2 cup purple cabbage
2 cups corn

1 large tomato
1 tablespoon lemon juice
1 tablespoon balsamic vinegar
1/4 teaspoon grated ginger

Chop and sauté garlic, onions, and celery. Chop the carrots, cabbage and tomato and mix together with the lemon juice, balsamic vinegar and ginger. Cut the pepper lengthwise and remove the seeds. Fill the peppers with vegetable mixture and bake in the over at 400 degrees for 25 minutes.

Make the dish Mexican by using cumin, paprika and chili powder in the place of the lemon, balsamic and ginger.

QUINOA AND MUSTARD SEEDS

This dish has a wonderful Indian flavor.

2 cups quinoa
1 onion
2 tomatoes
2 tablespoons mustard seeds
1 teaspoon cumin
1 teaspoon dried ginger
1/4 teaspoon turmeric
Salt to taste
Olive oil
Fresh cilantro

Cook quinoa by first washing the quinoa by placing it in a fine mesh strainer and running cold water over the seeds for a few minutes. Then add two cups of water and the quinoa to a saucepan and bring to a boil, let simmer for 20 minutes. Chop the onions and tomatoes into small pieces. In a large skillet, place the mustard seeds and a little bit of olive oil, let the seeds sizzle for a minute or two and then add in onion and cook until tender. Add in the rest of the ingredients and stir and then mix together with the cooked quinoa. Top with fresh cilantro.

QUINOA CASSEROLE

1 cup quinoa
1/4 cup dried currants or raisons
1/4 cup sunflower seeds
1 cup celery
2 carrots
1 zucchini
1 or 2 bay leaves
1 tsp ground coriander
1/2 tsp paprika
1/2 tsp ground ginger
1/2 tsp ground cumin
Pinch of cinnamon
Olive oil
Salt and pepper to taste

Cook quinoa by first washing quinoa and then adding two cups of water and the quinoa to a saucepan and bring to a boil, let simmer for 20 minutes. Stir fry the vegetables in a bit of olive oil until lightly cooked. Add the vegetable mixture to the cooked quinoa and spices. Serve warm or cold.

LENTIL BURGERS

In these burgers, lentils are used instead of pinto or black beans.

1 cups brown lentils
2-4 cups water
3/4 cups sunflower seeds
1/2 medium red onion
1/8 cup nutritional yeast
2 tablespoons soy sauce
2 teaspoons cumin
1 cloves garlic

1 teaspoon paprika
Olive oil
Salt and pepper to taste

Cover lentils in water and bring to a boil, simmer at medium to low heat for an hour until thoroughly cooked. Drain lentils and place in a bowl and mash with a potato masher. Saute onion, garlic and pepper in olive oil until tender and then place in the bowl. Add sunflower seeds and spices. Form the mixture into individual patties and then place on a non-stick pan and cook at 350 degrees for 20 minutes or until done.
Try with cayenne pepper for that extra zing.

CABBAGE ROLL-UPS

These simple cabbage roll-ups are surprisingly filling.

1 large cabbage leaf
1/2 avocado mashed
Salsa to flavor
Chopped sprouts (alfalfa, broccoli, bean...)

A cabbage leaf makes a great sandwich for any filling. Try softening the cabbage first by letting in soak in a bowl of warm water for a few minutes and then pat dry. What should you put inside? Try any of the burger recipes, hummus, fresh vegetables (red peppers, onions, broccoli) or just avocado and salsa. The combinations are endless.

TWICE-BAKED POTATOES

We use Yukon potatoes for this dish, but you can use any potatoes you like.

6-8 large potatoes
1 cup fresh or frozen corn
1 medium yellow onion
1 cup green beans, chopped
1 teaspoon ground garlic
Salt and pepper to taste

Bake potatoes in the oven at 350 degrees for 45 minutes to an hour. Let potatoes cool for a while and then cut lengthwise and scoop out the insides. Mix potatoes with the vegetables and spices and then fill the potato skins with mixture. Place on a cookie sheet and bake for another 20 minutes. The variations on this recipe are endless, try using other vegetables such as lima beans, peas, carrots or whatever vegetable your family enjoys.

DESSERT

All of the following sorbets and nice creams can be made two ways. The first is to mix the ingredients and then use an ice cream maker to make them smooth. The second is to use ice cubes or frozen fruit and simply blend and serve.

FRUIT SORBET

The ripest fruits are the best. Pick two cups of each fruits you have available. Try these combinations:

Watermelon (without seeds) and mangos
Strawberry banana
Cranberry and pear
Banana pineapple

Blend in blender until smooth and then freeze using an ice cream machine. Let it soften a bit before eating.

BANANA NICE CREAM

Here is a nice, quick treat.

2 frozen bananas
1 cup rice, coconut or almond milk
2 tablespoons smooth almond butter

Blend in blender or food processer until smooth, serve right away.

AVOCADO AND CHOCOLATE

As strange as this may sound, it is a traditional dish is areas of the world where avocados grow. If you are really trying to lose weight, you should avoid avocados, but as an occasional treat this isn't too bad.

2 large soft avocados
2 cups dark unsweetened chocolate
1/8 cup coconut milk
1 T vanilla extract
Frozen raspberries
1 T orange juice

Blend in blender or food processer until smooth, serve right away.

CHOCOLATE QUINOA

I found this recipe on line at a great blog called Green Lite Bites (www.greenlitebites.com). I've changed it a bit to fit our experiments; give it a try!

1/4 cup dry quinoa rinsed
1/2 cup chocolate soy or coconut milk

1 tablespoon unsweetened cocoa powder
1/2 teaspoon almond extract

Place all ingredients into a pan and cover. Lightly boil for 15 minutes in a covered pan until quinoa is cooked. Try it with fresh berries or nuts.

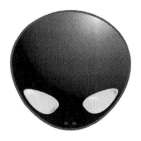

RESOURCES

I'm hoping that this is not the end of your journey, but the start. Here are some great resources to continue on your way.

You can find a Naturopathic doctor in your area to help you with all of your health concerns by going to the American Association of Naturopathic Physicians website: www.naturopathic.org

WEB

This book has its own website where you can meet other people on the journey, get more tips, ask questions and do battle with aliens: www.thealiendiet.com

You can also find me at my blog: www.olsonnd.com

I have a page for this book and there is a group on Facebook where you can join in the conversation, ask questions, and get support for making lifestyle changes.

BOOKS

Breaking the Food Seduction by Neal Barnard MD (St. Martins' Griffin Press, 2003). This book covers the addictive qualities of many of the foods that we eat.

Eat to Live, by Joel Fuhrman MD (Little, Brown and Company, 2003). This book is a classic even though it has only been around for a few years. Pick this up and read it, it will change your life.

Omnivore's Dilemma, by Michael Pollan (Penguin Press, 2007). This is a great read for anyone interested in health and where our food comes from.

Prevent and Reverse Heart Disease, by Caldwell B Esselstyn. (Avery Press, 2007). This is a great book about how cholesterol levels are tied closely to overall heart health and how a plant-based diet can reverse heart disease.

Sugarettes, by Scott Olson ND (BookSurge Publishing, 2008). This is my book that covers the damage and the addicting qualities of sugar.

The Botany of Desire: A Plant's Eye View of the World, by Michael Pollan (New York: Random House Press, 2001).

The China Study, by Colin Campbell (Benbella Books, 2006). The China Study is a landmark study reinforcing the idea that we need to eat many more plants than we currently do.

The Engine 2 Diet, by Rip Esselstyn (Wellness Central, 2009). Rip has popularized a plant-based diet showing that people can lose dramatic weight and improve their health when they follow a vegan diet.

COOKBOOKS

Ani's Raw Food Essentials, by Ani Phyo (Da Capo Lifelong Books, 2010)

Ani's Raw Food Desserts: 85 Easy, Delectable Sweets and Treats, by Ani Phyo (Da Capo Lifelong Books, 2009)

Green for Life by Victoria Boutenko (Raw Family Publishing, 2005)

The Vegan Table: 200 Unforgettable Recipes for Entertaining Every Guest at Every Occasion by Colleen Patrick-Goudreau (Fair Winds Press, 2009)

The World Goes Raw Cookbook by Lisa Mann (Square One Publishers, 2010)

Veganomicon: The Ultimate Vegan Cookbook by Isa Chandra Moskowitz and Terry Hope Romero (Da Capo Lifelong Books, 2007)

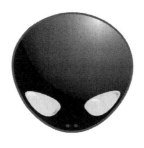

APPENDIX A

HOW TO EXERCISE

I put this how-to-exercise guide in the back of the book because exercising for weight loss can be surprisingly technical. If writing this section puts the author to sleep, then it cannot be too much fun for the reader. Make sure you check out the "Make it Simple" section below if your eyes start crossing when you read this.

How to exercise is important information because what many people call exercise won't help you lose weight. People often don't take their exercise routines seriously enough or work hard enough to really impact their weight. When you are ready (and have had enough coffee) wade through the rest of this section to discover how you should be exercising if you want to super-charge your weight loss. First, let me give you the short formula for weight-loss-inspiring exercise:

- You need to exercise aerobically in a sustained way at 70 percent of maximum.
- You need to strength train at 70 percent of your maximum.

Let's break those sentences down so we can understand what they mean.

AEROBIC SUSTAINED EXERCISE AT 70 PERCENT OF MAXIMUM

For weight loss, you need to perform a very specific type of exercise: a *sustained aerobic exercise where you are working at 70 percent or more of maximum.*

AEROBIC EXERCISE

Aerobic exercise is the easiest to explain. It is the type of exercise that causes your heart rate to increase and you start breathing hard. Aerobic exercises are what you think about when you hear the word "exercise" (walking, running, cycling, playing, and most sports). Non-aerobic exercises are those (like weight lifting) where your breathing doesn't have to increase for you to participate in them. The difference between the two is that your body needs more oxygen when you start off running (aerobic), but it doesn't need oxygen to lift those heavy weights (non-aerobic).

SUSTAINED EXERCISE

Sustained exercises seem pretty simple; they are exercises during which your heart rate is up at a target range (I'll explain that later) for an extended period. Exercises such as running or jogging, jumping rope, cross-country skiing, walking (once again in target heart range), running in place, bicycling, rowing, swimming, stair climbing, and dancing can all be sustained exercises.

Stop-and-go exercises do not count. Stop-and-go exercises include tennis, downhill skiing, football, racquetball or handball.

basketball, soccer, weight lifting, sprinting, golf, and many more. This is not to say that these exercises are not good for you (they are), but if you are going to be spending time exercising to lose weight you might as well be spending your time correctly.

Many people will say that they get enough exercise doing housework, or chasing the kids around the house, or that they work in a job like construction that is physically demanding. However, even though these exercises increase your heart rate, they are more like the stop-and-go exercises and have less of a benefit for weight loss.

The key to sustained exercise is that your heart rate is increased for a long period of time and there is not a time when you are pausing and your heart rate drops.

70 PERCENT OF MAXIMUM

What the heck is "70 percent of maximum"? This is a way to measure how hard you are working when you exercise. Study after study has shown that exercise intensity is a key ingredient to both increasing metabolism and exercising for weight loss.

While there are many ways to measure the intensity of a workout, the easiest way is to buy a heart rate monitor. Heart rate monitors have become cheap and easy to use over the last few years. Many machines like treadmills or elliptical trainers have heart rate monitors built in. In order to lose weight and boost your metabolism you need to exercise at least 70 percent of your maximum heart rate.

DETERMINING YOUR SEVENTY PERCENT OF MAXIMUM

To find out what your 70 percent of maximum is, you first you have to find out your maximum heart rate. When you have your maximum heart rate, you can then determine 70 percent from that amount.

To find your target heart rate, use this simple formula: subtract your age from the number 220. The result of your calculation is a good estimation of your Maximum Heart Rate. Now that you have your Maximum Heart Rate, you can compute your 70 percent (if you don't remember how to do this math, you simply take the number and times it by .70).

> **For example**: a forty-five-year-old's Maximum Heart Rate is 175 (220 minus 45). From the maximum heart rate you can compute 70 percent to find your recommended training level for the optimal workout level. For our forty-five-year-old, this would be 122 (175 x .70) beats per minute or more.

Our forty-five-year-old would want to make sure that when she is exercising her heart rate is above 122 beats per minute the whole time.

DURATION

How long should you exercise? Most research shows that you should be exercising at least 30 minutes a day if you are exercising every day (or around 150-200 minutes a week).[54]

MAKE IT SIMPLE

If you are the type of person who reads the previous paragraphs and their brain freezes, then this section is for you.

What you need to know about the previous sections is that if you are going to exercise then you need to work hard. This is not to suggest that you push yourself to your limits, but that you exercise at a pretty good rate. The question is: How do you know that you are working at a pretty good rate if you don't have a heart rate monitor or don't want to perform calculus? Try this: The Breath Method.

Imagine that you have chosen walking as your exercise. You want to walk intensely enough to where it is difficult but not impossible to carry on a conversation. This method works fairly well as long as you continue to pay attention the whole time. Many heart rate monitors can be set to beep if you get below a certain heart rate; you won't have that.

When you choose the breath method, the tendency is to slow down without even noticing it. So, use the breath method if you want to but make sure you keep the amount of effort up during the whole exercise period. I don't use a heart rate monitor and have learned over time what it feels like to exercise in this range. You too will get a feel for it and won't need to pay as much attention.

The key to all of this is to *exercise* when you are exercising and not just go out for a casual stroll. If you really want to turn the tables on your slow metabolism, you have to pick up your intensity.

PUTTING AEROBIC EXERCISE TOGETHER

Okay, now you know how intense your exercise should be and you know that it needs to be a sustained type of exercise. But how long and how often should you exercise?

For weight loss, you need to exercise for at least forty minutes to one hour every time you work out. This is the amount of time it takes to both boost your metabolism and make an impact on your weight loss.

Some of the research has shown that the boost to metabolism will last up to forty-eight hours, so you should consider doing aerobic exercise at least every other day. Doing aerobic exercise one day and strength training the other day is a great alternative for many people. Although, doing your aerobic exercise every day (or at least five times a week) will have the most benefit. Once again, start where you are and do what you can. If you can only walk around the block then that is your exercise.

As you are doing the whole program, the diet and exercise start to work together. The more weight you lose, the better you will feel, and the more exercise you can do. This leads to more weight loss and feeling even better and being able to exercise even more.

STRENGTH EXERCISE

I know that this is the last thing that you want to hear, but you also need to add weight lifting or strength training to your exercise program. Strength training builds muscles and, remember, the more muscle mass you have the higher your BMR. Muscles are some of the most metabolically active tissue you have. More muscle mass means more calories burned even when you are sleeping; you feel better; you keep your weight down; and you may live a longer and healthier life.

Adding a weight-lifting program is one of the essentials of a good weight-loss strategy. Find a personal trainer who understands these concepts and get started in a weight-lifting program. A personal trainer can help you to set goals and stick with them. It is best to start out slow and then build as you go along.

Two or three weight-lifting sessions a week are ideal. Some people will do a little every day (each day focusing on a different body part). Whatever works for you: Choose it and Do it. The payoff for adding weight lifting to your program is great. You will feel wonderful.

70 PERCENT OF MAXIMUM... AGAIN?

Is this starting to sound familiar? I don't know how to explain it, but there is something about how intensely you work out that supercharges your metabolism. So, just like the aerobic exercise section above, when you strength train, you want to work out at 70 percent of maximum.

Unlike using your heart rate to measure your 70 percent of maximum for aerobic exercise, when you strength train, your 70 percent of maximum has to do with how much you can lift in a single lift and, as you get stronger, your 70 percent of maximum will change. If you are not familiar with weight lifting, I would suggest that you have a personal trainer help you out with your routine.

Seventy percent of maximum for strength training means that you determine the maximum you can lift on a certain lift or a certain machine and then you exercise at 70 percent of that for eight to ten repetitions.

> **For example**: Let's say you have determined the most you can lift doing leg extensions on a machine is 125 pounds. When you return to that machine, you want to lift 95 pounds (70 percent of 125 is 95 pounds). You want to lift this amount ten times, and you want to do this specific exercise three different times before moving on to the next muscle group.

With weight training, you don't want to start out lifting 70 percent of maximum; just start lifting weights. Once you are familiar with the equipment and you have begun building muscle, then start lifting heavier amounts.

FOCUS ON LARGE MUSCLES

In order to be able to really see a difference in weight loss, you want to focus your strength training on the large muscle groups in your body. The legs contain some of the largest muscles in your body, but you can also do the large muscles of the arms.

You can strength train every other day, but if you lift weights three to five times a week that is enough for most people. If you are strength training every other day, you might want to do arms one day and legs the next day, or split up the exercises to best fit your routine.

As with any exercise, start slowly and build slowly. Remember: The first few times you go to the gym, you might just want to familiarize yourself with the machines and only do a few repetitions.

Summing it all up

Here is what you want to remember about exercising for weight loss:

- You need to exercise aerobically in a sustained way at 70 percent of maximum for at least 40 minutes every other day.

- You need strength train at 70 percent of your maximum two to three times a week.

- Try the breath method if you don't like gadgets or calculations.

- Always start slow and build.

- Your body will love you for working so hard!

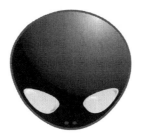

APPENDIX B

You may have noticed that there is an ND after my name and not an MD. The ND stands for Naturopathic Doctor. I'm often asked what kind of doctor a Naturopath is so here is an explanation:

NATUROPATHS: THE DOCTORS OF THE FUTURE

After being shuttled in and out of a doctor's appointment in less than 10 minutes with nothing but a prescription to show for it, you might be wishing for something better. You may have also wished that your doctor could not only prescribe the drugs you need, but also talk to you about what you can do to heal yourself using diet, nutrition, herbs, vitamins, and homeopathy, or other natural healing methods. Maybe, you think, the doctor of the future will have a more balanced approach and be your partner in health.

The doctor of the future is already here.

Naturopathic Doctors (NDs), who have attended licensed naturopathic colleges, have an understanding of both standard medical practice and natural healing methods. NDs are doctors who are trained very similarly to medical doctors but who have an entirely different approach to health and healing. Their approach recognizes the self-healing potential inside all of us. Naturopaths have the ability to help you decide between either medical or natural healing choices depending on your situation. Naturopaths work to uncover the root cause of the disease and not simply mask the problem by making symptoms go away with drug therapy.

Naturopaths recognize that there are many routes to health including exercise, diet, digestion, and elimination and they use natural healing methods such as herbs, vitamins, homeopathy, nutrition and much more. In short, naturopathic doctors treat the whole person. Naturopathic doctors take the time to educate the patient both on their disease and on ways to become healthier. They recognize that preventing diseases is often much easier than treating them.

While there currently aren't many naturopaths our numbers are growing. The licensing of Naturopaths is different in each state so they may not be able to prescribe drugs or perform certain procedures depending on which state you are in.

You can find a Naturopathic doctor in your area to help you with all of your health concerns by going to the American Association of Naturopathic Physicians website: www.naturopathic.org

[ENDNOTES]

1   Rajendrakumar Patel, MD, Rakesh Sarma, MD, Edwin GrimsleyE: Popular sweetener sucralose as a migraine trigger. Headache. 2006 Sep;46(8):1303-4.

2   Food Chemical News, June 12, 1995, Page 27.

3   Lavin JH, French SJ, Read NW: The effect of sucrose- and aspartame-sweetened drinks on energy intake, hunger and food choice of female, moderately restrained eaters. Int J Obes Relat Metab Disord. 1997 Jan;21(1):37-42.

4   Remig V, Franklin B, Margolis S, et al. Trans fats in America: a review of their use, consumption, health implications, and regulation. J Am Diet Assoc. 2010 Apr;110(4):585-92.

5   Kulkarni P, Getzenberg RH. High-fat diet, obesity and prostate disease: the ATX-LPA axis? Nat Clin Pract Urol. 2009 Mar;6(3):128-31.

6   Kaufman LN, Peterson MM, Smith SM. Hypertension and sympathetic hyperactivity induced in rats by high-fat or glucose diets. Am J Physiol. 1991 Jan;260(1 Pt 1):E95-100.

7   Riccardi G, Giacco R, Rivellese AA. Dietary fat, insulin sensitivity and the metabolic syndrome. Clin Nutr. 2004 Aug;23(4):447-56.

8   Osei K, Cottrell DA, Orabella MM.Insulin sensitivity, glucose effectiveness, and body fat distribution pattern in non-diabetic offspring of patients with NIDDM. Diabetes Care. 1991 Oct;14(10):890-6.

9   Granholm AC, Bimonte-Nelson HA, Moore AB, et al. Effects of a saturated fat and high cholesterol diet on memory and hippocampal morphology in the middle-aged rat. J Alzheimers Dis. 2008 Jun;14(2):133-45.

10   Brinkman MT, Baglietto L, Krishnan K, et a. Consumption of animal products, their nutrient components and postmenopausal circulating steroid hormone concentrations. Eur J Clin Nutr. 2010 Feb;64(2):176-83. Epub 2009 Nov 11.

11   Prentice RL, Caan B, Chlcbowski RT, Patterson R, et al. Low-fat dietary pattern and risk of invasive breast cancer: the Women's Health Initiative Randomized Controlled Dietary Modification Trial. JAMA. 2006 Feb 8;295(6):629-42.

12   Kohlmeier L, Simonsen N, van 't Veer P, Strain JJ, et al. Adipose tissue trans fatty acids and breast cancer in the European Community Multicenter Study on Antioxidants, Myocardial Infarction, and Breast Cancer. Cancer Epidemiol Biomarkers Prev. 1997 Sep;6(9):705-10.

13   Teng KT, Voon PT, Cheng HM, Nesaretnam K. Effects of Partially Hydrogenated, Semi-Saturated, and High Oleate Vegetable Oils on Inflammatory Markers and Lipids.Lipids. 2010 May 1.

14   Gaysinskaya VA, Karatayev O, Chang GQ, Leibowitz SF. Increased caloric intake after a high-fat preload: relation to circulating triglycerides and orexigenic peptides. Physiol Behav. 2007 May 16;91(1):142-53.

15   Shrapnel WS, Calvert GD, Nestel PJ, Truswell AS. Diet and coronary heart disease. The National Heart Foundation of Australia. Med J Aust. 1992 May 4;156 Suppl:S9-16.

16   Brunham LR, Kruit JK, Hayden MR, Verchere CB. Cholesterol in beta-cell dysfunction: the emerging connection between HDL cholesterol and type 2 diabetes. Curr Diab Rep 2010 Feb;10(1):55-60.

17   T. Colin Campbell. The China Study. Benbella Books, Dallas, TX, 2006.

18   Castelli WP. Making practical sense of clinical trial data in decreasing cardiovascular risk. Am J Cardiol. 2001 Aug 16;88(4A):16F-20F.

19   Fulgoni VL 3rd. Current protein intake in America: analysis of the National Health and Nutrition Examination Survey, 2003-2004. Am J Clin Nutr. 2008 May;87(5):1554S-1557S.

20   Protein and amino acid requirements in human nutrition, Report of a joint FAO/WHO/UNU Expert Consultation (WHO Technical Report Series ; no. 935) Geneva, World Health Organization, 2007.

21   Fung TT, van Dam RM, Hankinson SE, et al. Low-carbohydrate diets and all-cause and cause-specific mortality: two cohort studies. Ann Intern Med. 2010 Sep 7;153(5):289-98.

22   Casagrande SS, Wang Y, Anderson C, Gary TL. Have Americans increased their fruit and vegetable intake? The trends between 1988 and 2002. Am J Prev Med. 2007 Apr;32(4):257-63.

23   Kimmons J, Gillespie C, Seymour J, Serdula M, Blanck HM. Fruit and vegetable intake among adolescents and adults in the United States: percentage meeting individualized recommendations. Medscape J Med. 2009;11(1):26.

24   Alonso A, de la Fuente C, Martín-Arnau AM, et al. Fruit and vegetable consumption is inversely associated with blood pressure in a Mediterranean population with a high vegetable-fat intake: the Seguimiento Universidad de Navarra (SUN) Study. Br J Nutr. 2004 Aug;92(2):311-9.

25   Slavícek J, Kittnar O, Fraser GE, et al. Lifestyle decreases risk factors for cardiovascular diseases. Cent Eur J Public Health. 2008 Dec;16(4):161-4.

26   Joshipura KJ, Hu FB, Manson JE, et al. The effect of fruit and vegetable intake on risk for coronary heart disease. Ann Intern Med. 2001 Jun 19;134(12):1106-14.

27   Freedland SJ, Aronson WJ. Dietary intervention strategies to modulate prostate cancer risk and prognosis. Curr Opin Urol. 2009 May;19(3):263-7.

28   Block G, Patterson B, Subar A. Fruit, vegetables, and cancer prevention: a review of the epidemiological evidence. Nutr Cancer. 1992;18(1):1-29.

29   Patterson RE, Cadmus LA, Emond JA, Pierce JP. Physical activity, diet, adiposity and female breast cancer prognosis: A review of the epidemiologic literature. Maturitas. 2010 Jan 22.

30   Giem P, Beeson WL, Fraser GE. The incidence of dementia and intake of animal products: preliminary findings from the Adventist Health Study. Neuroepidemiology. 1993;12(1):28-36.

31   Barnard ND, Cohen J, Jenkins DJ, et al. A low-fat vegan diet and a conventional diabetes diet in the treatment of type 2 diabetes: a randomized, controlled, 74-wk clinical trial. Am J Clin Nutr. 2009 May;89(5):1588S-1596S. Epub 2009 Apr 1.

32   Turner-McGrievy GM, Barnard ND, Scialli AR. A two-year randomized weight loss trial comparing a vegan diet to a more moderate low-fat diet. Obesity (Silver Spring). 2007 Sep;15(9):2276-81.

33   Bes-Rastrollo M, Martínez-González MA, Sánchez-Villegas A, et al. Association of fiber intake and fruit/vegetable consumption with weight gain in a Mediterranean population. Nutrition. 2006 May;22(5):504-11.

34   He K, Hu FB, Colditz GA, Manson JE, Willett WC, Liu S. Changes in intake of fruits and vegetables in relation to risk of obesity and weight gain among middle-aged women. Int J Obes Relat Metab Disord. 2004 Dec;28(12):1569-74.

35   Brown L, Rosner B, Willett WW, Sacks FM. Cholesterol-lowering effects of dietary fiber: a meta-analysis. Am J Clin Nutr. 1999 Jan;69(1):30-42.

36   Suzuki R, Rylander-Rudqvist T, Ye W, Saji S, Adlercreutz H, Wolk A. Dietary fiber intake and risk of postmenopausal breast cancer defined by estrogen and progesterone receptor status–a prospective cohort study among Swedish women. Int J Cancer. 2008 Jan 15;122(2):403-12.

37   Liu S, Willett WC, Manson JE, et al. Relation between changes in intakes of dietary fiber and grain products and changes in weight and development of obesity among middle-aged women. Am J Clin Nutr. 2003 Nov;78(5):920-7.

38   Spangler R, Wittkowski KM, Goddard NL, et al: Opiate-like effects of sugar on gene expression in reward areas of the rat brain. Brain Res Mol Brain Res. 2004 May 19;124(2):134-42.

39   Galic MA, Persinger MA: Voluminous sucrose consumption in female rats: increased "nippiness" during periods of sucrose removal and possible oestrus periodicity. Psychol Rep. 2002 Feb;90(1):58-60.

40   Avena NM, Bocarsly ME, Rada P, et al: After daily bingeing on a sucrose solution, food deprivation induces anxiety and accumbens dopamine/acetylcholine imbalance. Physiol Behav. 2008 Jun 9;94(3):309-15.

41   Gosnell BA. Sucrose intake predicts rate of acquisition of cocaine self-administration. Psychopharmacology (Berl). 2000 Apr;149(3):286-92.

42   Colantuoni C, Schwenker J, McCarthy J, et al: Excessive sugar intake alters binding to dopamine and mu-opioid receptors in the brain. Neuroreport. 2001 Nov 16;12(16):3549-52.

43   Colantuoni C, Rada P, McCarthy J, et al: Evidence that intermittent, excessive sugar intake causes endogenous opioid dependence. Obes Res. 2002 Jun;10(6):478-88.

44   Drewnowski A, Krahn DD, Demitrack MA, et al. Taste responses and preferences for sweet high-fat foods: evidence for opioid involvement. Physiol Behav. 1992 Feb;51(2):371-9.

45   Hazum E, Sabatka JJ, Chang KJ, et al. Morphine in cow and human milk: could dietary morphine constitute a ligand for specific morphine (mu) receptors? Science. 1981 Aug 28;213(4511):1010-2.

46   Smit HJ, Blackburn RJ. Reinforcing effects of caffeine and theobromine as found in chocolate. Psychopharmacology (Berl). 2005 Aug;181(1):101-6. Epub 2005 Oct 15.

47   di Tomaso E, Beltramo M, Piomelli D. Brain cannabinoids in chocolate. Nature. 1996 Aug 22;382(6593):677-8.

48   Ifland JR, Preuss HG, Marcus MT, et al. Refined food addiction: a classic substance use disorder. Med Hypotheses. 2009 May;72(5):518-26.

49   Williamson DL, Kirwan JP. A single bout of concentric resistance exercise increases basal metabolic rate 48 hours after exercise in healthy 59-77-year-old men. J Gerontol A Biol Sci Med Sci. 1997 Nov;52(6):M352-5.

50   Hunter GR, Byrne NM, et al. Increased resting energy expenditure after 40 minutes of aerobic but not resistance exercise. Obesity (Silver Spring). 2006 Nov;14(11):2018-25.

51   Hegsted DM. Calcium and osteoporosis. J Nutr. 1986 Nov;116(11):2316-9.

52   Hegsted DM. Fractures, calcium, and the modern diet. Am J Clin Nutr. 2001 Nov;74(5):571-3.

53   Muldoon MF, Manuck SB, Matthews KA.Lowering cholesterol concentrations and mortality: a quantitative review of primary prevention trials. BMJ. 1990 Aug 11;301(6747):309-14.

54   Chambliss HO. Exercise duration and intensity in a weight-loss program. Clin J Sport Med. 2005 Mar;15(2):113-5.

Made in the USA
Lexington, KY
06 February 2012